Coping with

SCOLIOSIS

Bettijane Eisenpreis

THE ROSEN PUBLISHING GROUP, INC./NEW YORK

To Steven, Alice, Elliot, and all the others who encouraged me to write this book and put up with my moods during the many months when I was laboring over it.

Published in 1998 by The Rosen Publishing Group, Inc.
29 East 21st Street, New York, NY 10010

Cover Photo © Custom Medical Stock Photo, Inc.; pp. 93, 95 © Novartis Pharmaceuticals Corporation

First Edition

Library of Congress Cataloging-in-Publication Data

Eisenpreis, Bettijane.
    Coping with scoliosis / Bettijane Eisenpreis. —1st ed.
      p.   cm.
    Includes bibliographical references and index.
    Summary: Defines and describes scoliosis, discussing how it is
diagnosed and treated and providing advice and resources for those
having this condition.
    ISBN 0-8239-2557-9
    1. Scoliosis—Juvenile literature. 2. Scoliosis in children—
Juvenile literature. 3. Spine—Abnormalities—Juvenile literature.
[1. Scoliosis.]   I. Title.
RJ482.S3E36 1999
616.7'3—dc21   98-37198
                                     CIP
                                     AC

Manufactured in the United States of America

About the Author

Bettijane Eisenpreis describes herself as a "word person." She enjoys the challenge of writing about health issues in consumer-friendly terms. "Medical professionals need and want to get their message across, but sometimes consumers don't understand technical language," she says. "That's where I come in."

As principal of Bettijane Eisenpreis, Writer-Editor-Public-Relations, Bettijane has written on a variety of medical topics, as well as helping others convey their messages. Her first book, *Coping: A Young Woman's Guide to Breast Cancer Prevention*, was published by Rosen Publishing in 1997. That book, like this one, was based on her personal experience as well as interviews with medical professionals, consumer advocates, and patients.

Working independently gives Bettijane an opportunity to enjoy New York City, where she lives next door to her son, Steven. She also loves to travel.

Acknowledgments

My special thanks go to Dr. John P. Lubicky, M.D., Chief of Staff of the Chicago Unit, Shriners Hospitals for Crippled Children, and Professor of Orthopedic Surgery, Rush Medical College. Thanks also to Randal R. Betz, M.D., Assistant Chief of Staff and Medical Director of the Spinal Cord Injury Unit, Shriners Hospital for Crippled Children, Philadelphia Unit.

I want to acknowledge the invaluable cooperation of a number of individuals associated with the Department of Orthopedic Surgery of St. Vincent's Medical Center in New York City. These include Thomas Haher, M.D., Chairman of Orthopedics; Steven A. Caruso, M.E., Director of Biomedical Engineering; Areta

Podhorodecki, M.D., Physical Medicine and Rehabilitation; and Marisela Gonzalez, Physical Therapist. Michael Neuwirth, M.D., author of *The Scoliosis Handbook* and Chief of Spine Services at the Hospital for Joint Diseases in New York City was kind enough to grant me a face-to-face interview.

My thanks to Roger Rosen of the Rosen Publishing Group for encouraging me to investigate some less traditional approaches to scoliosis. His suggestion led me to Bobbie Fultz, who not only answered my questions about yoga but became my teacher and friend. Thanks also to Sean Gallagher, P.T., Director, and Elyssa Rosenberg, Associate Director, of the Pilates Studio®, and Mary Newell, Feldenkrais Practitioner.

Carla Podzius, M.S.W., and John Podzius, Ph.D., were very generous in sharing their time and thoughts on the psychological aspects of coping with scoliosis with me, and I thank them.

My heartfelt gratitude goes to Joe O'Brien of the National Scoliosis Foundation; Janice Sacks of the Scoliosis Association, Inc.; and JoEllen Hegmann, President of the Scoliosis Association of Long Island. JoEllen answered my questions and put me in contact with the teenagers whose stories are central to this book. To them—Samantha, Christine, Danielle, Alicia, Sara, and Kristin—I want to say how much I enjoyed meeting you by phone and learning about your experiences. Thanks also to Michael Buff and Michelle Ann Mauney, whom I interviewed by phone, and Francesca Halter and Suzette Haden Elgin, Internet friends who consented to share their experiences.

Contents

Introduction

If, like me, you have lived with scoliosis a long time, you may think everyone knows about it. If you don't have it or have only recently heard the word, you may wonder why anyone would write a book about it. But I've discovered that many people don't know what it means; some who think they do, don't.

Since the beginning of medical history, doctors have known about scoliosis. Hippocrates, an ancient Greek physician known as the "father of medicine," named the condition on the basis of the Greek word for "crooked."

What is scoliosis? A short definition is "a sideways (lateral) curving of the spine, usually developing in late childhood or early adolescence." I had to cope with scoliosis as a teenager and that's why I'm writing this book. The treatment now is entirely different, and much better, than it was when I was a teen. But the emotions you experience when you find out you have scoliosis haven't changed a bit.

One of the hardest things about scoliosis is the age at which it is usually detected. Adolescence is a time of turmoil for even the most seemingly well-adjusted young people. During a relatively short period of time, tremendous changes are taking place in your life. Physically, you are changing from a child to an adult.

Along with these physical changes comes emotional

1

turmoil. One day you are content to be a child, happy and protected by adults, but the next day you can't wait to be free from restraints and treated like a grown-up. And the adults in your life—parents and teachers—are experiencing conflicts as well. They want you to "grow up," to "take responsibility," but they also want you to obey them—to accept the curfews and other limitations they impose "for your own good." Sometimes you feel as if you can't please anyone, least of all yourself.

Among the many conflicting feelings of adolescence is a desire to be like everyone else and fit in with friends. At the same time, you know that you are becoming a new person, a unique adult. Body image—the way you feel about the way you look—plays a prominent part in how you perceive yourself. You may want to look like your favorite athlete, a Hollywood celebrity, or someone in the senior class. If you think that you don't meet that ideal, and if that bothers you, you may feel bad about your body. Sadly, many teens do, even though their bodies are fine.

Scoliosis, by definition, poses a problem when it comes to body image. Your hips and shoulders may be uneven. And some curves may result in a hump on the center or one side of your back.

The fact that there is no physical pain associated with scoliosis, at least in the early stages, only makes matters more confusing. Most teens don't even know they have a problem until a doctor or teacher points it out.

My Own Story

If you are trying to cope with scoliosis, I know just how you feel. I also know that although scoliosis is a problem, it is one you can deal with. Dealing with scoliosis involves doing a number of things that will help make you a better adult—talking about your feelings, cooperating with your parents and other adults, making choices, and taking responsibility. While this may not be of much comfort, take my word for it: Coping with scoliosis can be a growth experience.

What I remember most about being a young teen was an intense desire to belong. I wanted to be just like the other girls. I wanted to be beautiful as defined by the standards of the time: blonde, blue-eyed, and possessing perfect features and a curvaceous figure. I wanted to excel in sports rather than in studies, to have lots of friends and boyfriends, and never to stay home on a Saturday night.

I hated the way I looked; I was skinny with dark hair and no "figure." My best features, my blue eyes, were obscured by glasses. No matter how hard I tried to look well groomed, I always felt my coat was buttoned wrong or my hair was straggly.

I thought that things could not possibly get worse, but when I was twelve, they did. When I was in seventh grade, we got a new gym teacher. Let's call her Miss Smith. She was young, dark-haired, slim, and very enthusiastic. She was not unkind to me. Probably she didn't notice me, since my principal occupation in gym class was trying to stay invisible.

One day, Miss Smith said she wanted to see me after class. My heart sank. After class, when she said that she needed to speak to my mother, I became even more fearful. I duly informed my mother that Miss Smith wanted to see her.

The day came, and the three of us met in Miss Smith's

office. As instructed, I came to the meeting wearing my gym clothes. The gym teacher showed my mother that one of my shoulders was higher than the other and one of my hips stuck out more prominently. It was easier to observe these differences when I was wearing a gym suit or a bathing suit. Miss Smith knew that many teenagers have scoliosis and was on the alert for any signs of the condition. She advised my mother to take me to the family doctor, who confirmed the diagnosis. I had scoliosis—a curvature of the spine.

Of course I felt awful. Now, in addition to not looking like Marilyn Monroe, I didn't look like anyone I knew. I became acutely aware that my shoulders and hips were uneven. I began to notice that my skirt hems were always crooked and I couldn't wear vertically striped dresses because the stripes all seemed to be pointing at my left knee. Horizontal stripes weren't much better. No matter how hard I tried to stand up straight, I couldn't.

This is only the beginning of my story. There was a happy ending. After treatment, my scoliosis was halted. I grew up, dated, married, had a child, and have had a very fulfilling career as a writer.

What Next?

At the time I learned I had it, a diagnosis of scoliosis was very rare, even though a sizable minority of people suffer from it. I was lucky because my condition was spotted early, when it could be treated. Early detection is important. Today, there are scoliosis screening programs in many public schools, and an increasing number of pediatricians check their patients for early signs. Still, the record is not perfect. Many children and adults still go untreated, often with painful results in later life. Many people think, erroneously, that "it isn't anything," or "it will go away."

This doesn't mean that everyone with scoliosis has to have treatment. In the majority of cases, watchful waiting is enough. According to the National Scoliosis Foundation, although one person in ten has scoliosis, only two or three in every thousand need active treatment; in one out of every thousand cases, surgery may be necessary.

If the curvature is spotted early, if it isn't bad, and if it doesn't get worse by the time you are eighteen or nineteen, then you can usually forget about it. While some adults develop severe scoliosis later in life, most do not.

This book discusses what scoliosis is and what it is not. The more information you have, the better you can deal with scoliosis, or its cousins, abnormal lordosis (swayback) and abnormal kyphosis (humpback). The book will then address how doctors diagnose scoliosis. You'll meet some young adults who were diagnosed with scoliosis, follow them through their treatment, and learn how they felt about it.

The rest of the book is about choices concerning treatment and lifestyle. Many of these choices will be yours, so you'll need to know the pros and cons. Should you wear a brace, and what kind? Should you have surgery? If so, when and what kind? Should you join a scoliosis support group, and how can you find one?

This book provides you with information but is not intended as a substitute for medical advice. It will give you a great deal of information to help you understand the choices confronting you. You don't have to make the decisions alone. You have your parents or other adults who are concerned with your well-being. If you work with them and let your wishes be known, things will probably work out well. You may even want to share part or all of this book with them.

If you have to make a decision about scoliosis, or if it appears to stand in the way of something you want, scoliosis may seem like the biggest obstacle in your life. But once you've learned the facts and vented your feelings and frustrations, you won't feel as intimidated by scoliosis. Arming yourself with knowledge and sharing your feelings are the greatest weapons against fear.

One day a few years ago, I was standing and talking with one of my older cousins, with whom I'm very close. Suddenly he said, "Bettijane, you're leaning to one side. Stand up straight!"

"Everett," I said, chuckling, "I would if I could, but I can't." He had known me since birth and had never realized that I had scoliosis!

If you have scoliosis, it's okay. The whole world is not watching. Everything really will be all right.

What Is Scoliosis?

In 1973, author Judy Blume, who is well known for her understanding of teenagers and their concerns, wrote *Deenie*, a book about a girl with scoliosis. This suggests that scoliosis was as important a topic for teens decades ago as it is today. Why?

Scoliosis is significant because it affects a part of the anatomy that, in some ways, defines us as human beings—the spine. Humans are part of a large class of animals called vertebrates, all of whom possess backbones. One trait that makes humans unique is the fact that we stand upright. This ability enabled humans (and other primates) to develop grasping thumbs. It also allowed for the development of a highly complex brain and nervous system. But this upright posture also puts the human spine under more stress than does the horizontal spine of other vertebrates.

To understand scoliosis and other spinal irregularities, we must first understand something about the spine itself.

The Backbone's Connected to the . . .

"The human body is more mechanical than anything I know," says Steven A. Caruso. Caruso was trained as a civil engineer and became the director of biomechanical engineering in the Department of Orthopedic Surgery at St.

Vincent's Medical Center in New York. He adds, "There is no system in the world more perfectly engineered than the human body."

Central to this perfectly engineered system, Caruso continues, is the spinal column. Although the word *column* may make you think of something straight and stiff, our spines aren't like that. They are flexible columns, made up of many different kinds of interlocking parts, which together allow us to move, bend, and lift.

The Vertebrae

The human spine is made up of twenty-four flexible pieces of bone called vertebrae; the sacrum; and the coccyx. The sacrum, which is the part of the spine that is connected to the pelvis, consists of five vertebrae that are fused together. The coccyx, or tailbone, is made up of an additional four fused vertebrae. The spine begins just below the head and ends with the coccyx (tailbone). It runs through a number of bodily regions, and its name changes along the way.

The uppermost section of the spine is the neck, or cervix. It is made up of seven vertebrae, known as the cervical vertebrae. Vertebrae are numbered from top to bottom. The neck vertebrae are C1 through C7.

Below the neck are the twelve upper spine vertebrae that support the ribs. They are located in the area of the chest, or thorax, from the Greek word for breastplate. These vertebrae are called the thoracic vertebrae, T1 through T12.

The lower, or lumbar, spine is composed of five vertebrae, L1 through L5. They are positioned just above the sacrum, which in turn sits atop the coccyx.

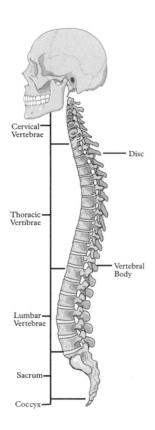

The human spine.

Beyond the Vertebrae

Between each vertebra and the one above it is a disc, a ring-shaped piece of cartilage with a fibrous outside and a jelly-like inside. The discs help cushion the spine against shocks and jolts. In addition, two facet joints connect each vertebra to the one above it. Together, the discs and facet joints make the spine strong and mobile. An intricate system of ligaments and muscles enables the individual pieces of the spine to move and connects them to other parts of the body.

9

Each vertebra has a hollow center, or vertebral canal. With the vertebrae joined together, these hollows form the spinal canal, through which the spinal cord runs. The spinal cord and the brain make up the body's central nervous system. It's like your own personal Internet, linking the central computer of the brain with sensors in the organs, arms, legs, skin, etc. Most of the time we take this mechanical marvel for granted. But when someone famous or close to us has an accident resulting in spinal injury or paralysis, we become acutely aware of the spine's vital role.

When someone has scoliosis, the spine is not straight. Not only the vertebrae and discs are affected; the whole spinal mechanism is thrown out of sync. Muscles and ligaments will be constricted on one side and overextended on the other, so they won't function normally.

Types of Spinal Deformities

If curvature of the spine is a deformity, does that mean a normal spine is absolutely straight? No. If you look at a person from the side, his or her upper spine should curve slightly backward, while curving forward at the waist area. However, it should be straight—give or take a few degrees—when you look at it from the back.

Scoliosis is not a disease, although it is sometimes caused by disease. It is one of several conditions called spinal deformities. This is a medical term. It doesn't mean that people with scoliosis are deformed. Many people with scoliosis are amazed at how few of their friends and relatives notice that one shoulder is higher than the other or that they appear to lean to one side. Some other spinal

Abnormal Lordosis

The normal front-to-back curve at the waist-line is called lordosis. Everybody is supposed to have it, to a degree. An abnormal lordosis, which causes the shoulders to sit too far back and the "butt" to stick out, is referred to as swayback. Not enough lordosis is flatback, which isn't normal, either.

deformities include abnormal lordosis, abnormal kyphosis, and Scheuermann's kyphosis.

Scoliosis

The simplest definition of scoliosis is a lateral, or side-to-side, curvature of the spine. If you look at the back of someone with scoliosis, you can't always see the curve beneath the skin and muscle, but you can see it on an X ray.

Scoliosis curves come in different patterns. The curve may take the shape of a C, or may be more gentle, like a parenthesis (. If a person has a C-curve, and if it is located in only one section of the spine, such as the thoracic or lumbar area, a second smaller, or compensating, curve may form in another section of the spine. In that case, because one part of the scoliosis is smaller than the other, it may look like a lopsided S.

11

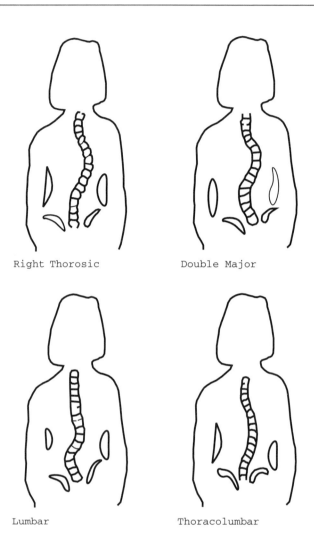

Right Thorosic   Double Major

Lumbar   Thoracolumbar

Some of the most common patterns of spinal curvatures.

The most common curve pattern is a right thoracic curve, a single C-curve located in the upper spine and bending toward the right. Other common curve patterns are thoracolumbar, a C-curve that starts in the chest area

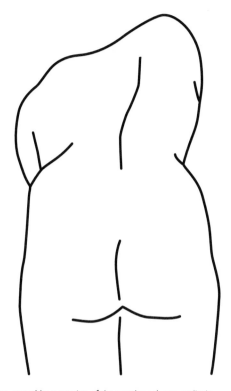

A typical rib hump caused by a rotation of the vertebrae due to scoliosis.

and ends below the waist; lumbar, a shorter C in the lower back; and double major, an S-curve whose two parts are roughly equal.

Often, when the spine curves to the side, the vertebrae move around, or rotate. This makes the ribs on the outside of the curve open up wide and the ribs on the inside of the curve grow closer together. The wide-open ribs form a "rib hump" on one side of the back. It becomes clearly visible when a scoliosis patient bends over.

Scoliosis is often invisible to the naked eye, especially

Abnormal Kyphosis

The normal sideways upper curve of the spine is kyphosis. When it is exaggerated, we say a person has an abnormal kyphosis, or round back. Abnormal kyphosis is often caused by unhealthy postural habits. Sitting and standing in abnormal positions can aggravate normal or slightly abnormal kyphosis, particularly during the adolescent growth period. This is especially true of girls, who grow faster than boys. Repeated slumping can develop into a permanent deformity. If caught in time, it may be cured by a back brace, but you can help prevent it altogether by maintaining good posture.

Scoliosis and abnormal kyphosis are sometimes confused because there are some similarities between them. If someone has a very pronounced rib hump, we may say this person has a kyphotic scoliosis. The main difference is that with scoliosis, the rib hump sticks out on one side and is more visible when a person bends over. An abnormal kyphosis shows up as a round, centered hump, whether a person is bending over or standing straight. Often the same treatment is used for both conditions.

when it starts in the teens. Because it can start small and progress rapidly as the child grows, it is important for doctors, teachers, and parents to know how to spot it. Not every scoliosis patient has a rib hump. Uneven shoulders and hips and slanting waistbands on skirts or pants can be telltale signs.

Structural vs. Nonstructural Scoliosis

Years ago, doctors thought that carrying books on the same side all the time gave children scoliosis. In most cases, this has not been found to be true, even though carrying heavy books on one side can lead to severe muscle strain and back pain.

Structural Scoliosis
Since carrying your books on one side has not been found to be a major cause of scoliosis, you might conclude that scoliosis is not simply the result of poor posture. And you'd be right most of the time. Most of the people who are referred to orthopedists (doctors concerned with deformities of the human skeleton) for treatment of spinal deformities have structural problems. Structural problems are difficulties, related to your spine's anatomy, that you have no control over. One sign of structural scoliosis is the presence of a rib hump.

Nonstructural Scoliosis
Sometimes, however, a person's spine will curve for a reason unrelated to the way his or her spine is formed, such as bad posture, illness, or injury. This type of scoliosis is

Scheuermann's Kyphosis

Abnormal kyphosis, or round back, is often postural in nature, but that is not always the case. Scheuermann's kyphosis was named for the doctor who first identified it in 1920, and experts are not sure what causes it. There are two main types of Scheuermann's kyphosis. The first is thoracic, which means it is located entirely in the upper spine area. This is a hereditary and progressive problem, but it is not painful. The thoracic type is mainly a problem for cosmetic (appearance) reasons. The second type of Scheuermann's kyphosis is dorsolumbar, or located in the waist and lower spine. Dorsolumbar kyphosis can be painful and may result from trauma or from too much pressure on an immature spine. It can be the result of athletic injuries and should be taken seriously. Sometimes pain persists and surgery is necessary to correct this condition.

called nonstructural scoliosis, and it may be temporary.

The most common form of nonstructural scoliosis is postural scoliosis. Unbalanced postures can become a habit. When a young person, whose body is still developing, sits with all her weight on one hip or stands with most of her weight on one leg, the muscles on one side of her trunk and hips may become more flexible, and the other side may tighten up. Over time the bone and soft tissue may be adapted to the new posture. Repeating unhealthy posture habits while you are growing really can affect the way your muscles and bones grow. Postural scoliosis can, in some cases, develop into structural scoliosis. This is why it's a good idea to develop a regular exercise routine early in life so that standing, walking, and sitting correctly will become natural.

A few other nonstructural causes of scoliosis are worth mentioning. Sometimes a person's legs either are or appear to be different lengths. This can be caused by an actual difference in the length of the bones, or by a dislocated hip. Also, deformities—either from birth or trauma (injury)—may make the pelvis higher on one side than the other. If one of these conditions causes one leg to be longer than the other, the spine may curve from side to side when the person stands up, although when he is sitting or lying down it is not truly curved. Our heads want to look straight ahead, at the horizon, and our bodies will do their best to compensate to achieve that goal. If you do correct the difference in leg length, will the spine snap back? Frequently, it will, especially if the leg problem was caused by something temporary, such as a dislocated hip. But if the body gets used to the condition, it may be harder to correct.

Another nonstructural problem that may cause the spine to curve is spasm in the back muscles due to injury. When you throw your back out and feel pain going down one leg, the muscles tighten up, causing the spine to shift away from the painful side. Usually, if the pain goes away, the spine straightens. This temporary curvature of the spine is not a true scoliosis.

Idiopathic Scoliosis

The great majority of scoliosis cases, perhaps as many as 80 to 90 percent, come under the heading of idiopathic, which means "having no known cause." That doesn't mean there isn't a cause, just that we don't know it at present. More research is needed.

There are four types of idiopathic scoliosis, based on the age that the patient was when the condition was first detected. Infantile idiopathic scoliosis, which appears between birth and the age of three, is not seen very often in the United States. It seems to be different in nature from juvenile or adolescent scoliosis. It is called idiopathic because doctors don't know what causes it, but they suspect the cause is not what causes juvenile or adolescent scoliosis.

The main difference between juvenile idiopathic scoliosis and the adolescent variety is that the juvenile type develops between the ages of three and ten and isn't quite as common. Although the curves seen in both may look similar, children with the juvenile variety are at greater risk of their curves progressing because they have more years of growth before them.

The most common type is adolescent idiopathic scoliosis, which appears at or near the time that puberty begins, between the ages of ten and thirteen. Before the days of school screening programs for scoliosis, adolescent scoliosis was often overlooked. It usually starts as a mild, hardly visible curvature. It is painless at first, which makes early detection doubly important, because it can be painful later on if left untreated.

18

Is adult idiopathic scoliosis any different? Probably not. It may be adolescent scoliosis that wasn't spotted earlier, or that was spotted but continued to progress after the end of adolescence. People used to think that curves couldn't progress after a person reached maturity, but that didn't prove true. Some adults get what is called degenerative scoliosis, caused by disease of the discs of the spine or arthritis in the facet joints. Sometimes it is hard to tell if scoliosis in an adult is degenerative or idiopathic.

Scoliosis with Known Causes

Although we don't know the cause of idiopathic scoliosis, a sizable minority of cases—about 15 percent—do have a known cause. By studying these cases, researchers are beginning to get some clues about the origins of idiopathic scoliosis.

For example, there is congenital scoliosis. Most people, hearing that a disease or condition is congenital, think that it is genetic or inherited. That's not always true. Congenital only means that you were born with it; it has nothing to do with where you got it. If a developing baby experiences a trauma in the womb, for example, some of its vertebrae can become malformed.

A malformed vertebra may be shaped like a wedge or triangle, called a "hemivertebra" because it is only half of a normal vertebra, or it may be like a block, in which the spaces between the vertebrae haven't formed. A vertebra affected by a congenital defect also can take the shape of a bar, where the spaces have formed on one side but the other side is solid. These misshapen vertebrae cause the spine to curve, resulting in scoliosis.

While congenital scoliosis is not necessarily genetic in origin, some scoliosis may be. An inherited disease of the connective tissue (ligaments and tendons) called Marfan syndrome, which also affects the heart and other organs, causes severe scoliosis in many patients. There are about 40,000 known cases of Marfan syndrome in the United States. Although it is a rare disease, it is a serious problem for those affected by it.

Idiopathic scoliosis seems to run in families, so physicians and researchers assume that genes play a part. The questions "Which genes?" and "What part do they play?" have not been answered. No one has found a scoliosis gene, and it is unlikely that they will. Researchers suspect that even if the cause of idiopathic scoliosis is genetic, the trait may be transmitted on several different genes, or a combination of genes. Genes seem to be one factor, but they are not the only one.

Some scoliosis is caused by diseases of the nervous system. When my scoliosis was diagnosed in the 1940s, the first thing the doctors asked me was, "Have you ever had a high fever without knowing the cause?" The Salk polio vaccine had not yet been developed, and many doctors assumed that someone who had scoliosis could have had polio at some point, even if it had not been diagnosed. This disease, which people used to call "infantile paralysis" (incorrectly—it affects adults as well as children), is a central nervous system infection that can result in paralysis of the muscles on one side of the body, causing the spine to curve. Thanks to the Salk vaccine, polio is seldom found in the United States today, but cerebral palsy—a birth defect resulting in damage to the nervous system—is still with us. It too can produce scoliosis as a result of muscle imbalance.

In fact, some doctors believe that most scoliosis has its roots in the nervous system. Dr. John Lubicky, chief of staff at the Shriners Hospitals for Crippled Children's Chicago Unit, told me, "Idiopathic scoliosis is probably a neurological disease. There are a number of studies that indicate that. There are some studies that show, for example, that people with scoliosis have an abnormal joint position sense or balance abnormalities." He continued, "There seems to be some problem with the righting mechanism [in people with scoliosis]; obviously, the neurological problem is not [prominent] enough in the average case of idiopathic scoliosis to recognize."

What's a "righting mechanism"? Remember those big, weighted plastic toys that sit on the floor, usually with a picture of a popular cartoon character on them? You punch them, and they bob back up to an upright position. That's a perfect example of a righting mechanism at work.

Scoliosis also can be caused by muscle diseases, such as muscular dystrophy, a usually hereditary disease marked by progressive muscular deterioration. Weak muscles cause imbalance in the spine, especially when the back is unsupported. When a child with muscular dystrophy is lying down, his or her spine may have almost no curvature, but when he or she stands up, the scoliosis may worsen dramatically.

Scoliosis may be a side effect of trauma to the body, such as fractured vertebrae, certain kinds of surgery, or radiation therapy. Sometimes radiation therapy, used to kill a cancerous tumor and save a child's life, can damage the "growth plates" at the end of the vertebrae and cause the spine to develop abnormally. These are not common causes of scoliosis, but they may give us some answers in the future.

Who Gets Scoliosis?

As you read further in this book, you may notice that most of the scoliosis patients I have interviewed are girls. When they are children, both boys and girls get scoliosis, but when they enter the teens, it is five to eight times more likely that a girl's spinal curves will increase and need treatment than a boy's.

Why this difference? We don't know, though many researchers think it has something to do with hormones. It may have to do with the fact that many girls experience the teenage "growth spurt" earlier than boys and achieve their full growth earlier. There are more questions about this than answers, but when we do find the answers, we may know what causes scoliosis and how to treat it.

At present, early detection is the key to controlling scoliosis before it becomes a major problem. How scoliosis is detected is the subject of the next chapter.

Spotting Scoliosis

School nurses were the ones who spotted scoliosis in Elizabeth, age eight, and Sara, age ten. The school doctor diagnosed Alicia's scoliosis; she was eleven at the time. Eleven-year-old Sara-Marie experienced mild backaches after gymnastics, so she went to an orthopedist, who discovered her curvature. For Samantha and Kristin, scoliosis was discovered by accident when they had chest X rays taken for bronchial infections. Michelle had open-heart surgery when she was four to correct a birth defect; at age six, a follow-up examination found that her heart was fine but revealed that she had scoliosis.

The Importance of Early Detection

These young women all have several things in common. Their scoliosis was detected and treated early. Today, all of them are leading healthy, normal lives. Their stories show the importance of early detection of scoliosis.

The Scoliosis Research Society estimates that about 10 percent of the adolescents in the United States (about 1 million teens) have scoliosis, but only a fourth of that group need any kind of treatment. If the curve is detected early, while it is still small (usually when a child is just entering adolescence), it can be more easily treated. Often the only treatment needed will be watchful waiting—observation by a doctor to make sure the curve does not progress. Or the doctor may observe the patient for a few months or a year and, if the curve does continue to progress, may prescribe a brace.

According to a 1993 study commissioned by the Scoliosis Research Society, bracing often can be effective in preventing progression of scoliosis in many cases, but only if the condition is detected early. So the sooner the better.

Looking at Yourself

Early detection is especially important for teens with a family history of scoliosis, but it's not limited to them. It might be a good idea to inspect yourself for scoliosis from time to time. There are a few clues you can check for.

First, stand in front of a mirror and look at yourself. Stand naturally, not at attention. Is one shoulder higher than the other? Do your hips appear to be uneven? For girls, do your breasts seem even, or does one look much larger than the other? A slight unevenness in breast size is normal, but in some cases of scoliosis the ribs on one side push one breast out so that it looks larger or more prominent than the other. In some fairly rare cases, you may feel a slight pain in your back. Don't ignore it; report it. If you do feel pain, it's important to see a doctor about it.

If you think you may have scoliosis, ask your mom, dad, or an older sibling to look at you from the back. While they are looking, bend over and touch your toes. If you have a rib hump, it will be more apparent when you're bending over than when you're standing up straight.

Even if you don't notice anything out of the ordinary, someone in the family may. Mothers have spotted slanting waistlines and uneven hems when shopping with their daughters for new school clothes. Or a son may complain of back pain that alerts parents to possible problems. Parents who have had scoliosis are especially alert to changes in their children's backs.

If you think you may have a curve, no matter how slight, it's important to call it to your parents' attention. They can apply some of the screening tests described in this chapter, and if there is any problem at all, they should bring it to the attention of your pediatrician or family doctor.

School Screening: Easy and Effective

The Scoliosis Research Society believes that school screening is the most effective tool for early detection. Still, some people question whether it pays to examine a whole school population when fewer than eighty of every one thousand children will have any degree of scoliosis. Some doctors wonder whether school screening programs produce too many "false positive" diagnoses and thus cause unnecessary anxiety. But while eighty out of one thousand sounds like a low number, it's a different story when you are one of the eighty.

There is legislation requiring scoliosis-screening programs in more than twenty-two states, with five or six more states encouraging school districts to conduct screening on a voluntary basis. Schools are where kids spend most of their time. It's easy to train school nurses or gym teachers to conduct these screenings. They don't take

25

much time, and many cases of scoliosis are spotted early this way. Like everything else, scoliosis screening must be done right to be effective.

The ages at which school screening programs are conducted vary, but ten to fourteen is the range recommended by the National Scoliosis Foundation, a patient advocacy group, and the Scoliosis Research Society, a group of orthopedic surgeons specializing in scoliosis. The American Academy of Orthopedic Surgeons says it's early enough to check girls when they are between the ages of eleven and thirteen, and boys at age thirteen or fourteen.

If you've already been examined for scoliosis at school, you know the drill. If your school doesn't have a program or you haven't reached the starting age yet, here's a general description of a typical screening program: The day before, a school nurse or public health official may tell you what's going to happen and what the screeners are looking for. He or she will explain what scoliosis is, stressing the fact that it's good to screen during early and mid-adolescence, when mild curvatures can often be stopped before they get worse. The talk will probably include a description of problems that can develop when scoliosis goes untreated, such as severe back pain, respiratory difficulties, and possible heart problems. You may get a chance to ask questions, if you have any.

During the exam itself, boys will be asked to wear something like gym shorts and girls will wear shorts and backless tops, such as bras or halters. First, you will be asked to stand, with your eyes facing straight ahead. Whoever is doing the exam—a nurse, a gym teacher, or sometimes a doctor—will be looking for asymmetry (unevenness). If your hips and shoulders don't line up, the waistline of your shorts ride up on one side, or your head seems to tilt to one side or the other, the examiner will make a note of it. It's important to stand in your natural posture so that if there is a problem, it will be found.

Then you will be asked to bend forward. You may be asked to bend over and touch your toes, or to put your hands together (as if you were going to dive) and lean forward. Both of these exercises are variations of the Adams Forward-Bend Test. If there's a rib hump caused by the rotation of the spine, it will be easier to see when you bend over. The rib hump is a good way to tell the difference between poor posture and a curvature of the spine. If your shoulders sag or slump because you don't always stand up straight, you probably won't have a rib hump.

Next you will be asked to stand up straight again, and the examiner will look at you from behind. If there's a curve in the upper (thoracic) spine, he or she may be able to see it with the naked eye. It's not enough just to look at the back, because there may be a curve in the lower spine or the curve may not be that obvious, so the examiner will also run a hand along your spine. While he or she is at it, the examiner will also look at you from the side to make sure that your spine curves in a gentle S, with a normal degree of kyphosis (forward bend) at the top and lordosis (outward bend) at the bottom.

Usually, that's all there is to it. Before you know it, you'll be back in your classroom. If you're a ten-year-old girl, you'll be checked again a few times during the coming years. Boys don't have to be checked as often because they reach puberty later and their spinal curves usually don't progress as much.

For most teens, that's it—end of story. But if you do have scoliosis, or the screener suspects that you might, you'll be told to see your own doctor—either the pediatrician or family doctor, or an orthopedist. A note will be sent home to your parents, or the school will call them.

But It Doesn't Hurt!

There's no pain with most idiopathic adolescent scoliosis, but that doesn't mean there won't be pain later, if the curve continues to progress. Our vertebrae were designed to sit squarely on top of each other, with the discs serving as neat little cushions between each one. If they don't fit right, the discs will get squeezed or displaced later in life, causing severe back pain. This displacement is frequently referred to as a slipped disc.

You may have heard people say, "Oh, my aching back!" Did you know that back pain is the largest cause of absences from work in the United States? The September 1996 issue of *Health* magazine reported that every year, half of all Americans of working age have at least one significant episode of lower back pain. The U.S. government has estimated that $25 billion is spent each year on health care for the approximately 80 million people who are suffering from back pain. So even though it's inconvenient and you may dread the prospect of wearing a brace, it's far better to take care of scoliosis now than later.

Other problems could develop later in life if scoliosis is not treated. When the spine curves, the ribs rotate, growing closer on one side and spreading farther apart on the other. This may result in the heart or lungs being squeezed. People with severe scoliosis sometimes have trouble breathing. Heart problems may result as well.

For girls, there used to be a concern that a lumbar (lower back) scoliosis would interfere with the expansion of the uterus in pregnancy, causing problems in childbirth. Actually, most women with scoliosis report that the childbirth itself goes fine, but if there is back pain from a slipped disc or other complications of scoliosis, it may get worse during pregnancy. The spine is required to carry a lot of extra weight at this time, so if there is a problem, pregnancy may aggravate it.

The risk of scoliosis to pregnancy was exaggerated in the past. But avoiding extra back pain later is one more reason to have scoliosis treated while you're young.

The Odds Are in Your Favor

The scoliosis screening is over. If you are in the vast majority of teens, you passed with flying colors. So that means you can relax, right? Well, almost.

First of all, it depends how old you are. You may have to go through the same ritual several times, and scoliosis may show up later, as your body continues to mature in early adolescence. Second, some curves do show up in adulthood, although the chances of this are slight if you have no curve during your teens.

The screening will make you more aware of how important it is to keep your back straight and strong. Good back care is part of an overall physical fitness program.

What do you do to stay healthy? Do you take part in gym class with enthusiasm, or are you like I was, trying to dream up excuses to be as inactive as possible? Does your school have a good physical education department, or was gym class a casualty of budget cuts? If so, there are other ways to exercise.

How about your diet? Are you eating well-balanced meals each day, with plenty of fruits and green vegetables? Are you getting lots of calcium—not in vitamin pills but in milk and dairy foods—to help build strong bones? It is important to eat well to maintain a healthy lifestyle.

If the Screening Indicates a Problem

What happens if you do have to take a note home saying you should see your doctor? For many of those screened, the only treatment prescribed by the doctor will be "watchful waiting." A few others will need more aggressive therapy.

If the doctor does say, "Let's wait and see what develops. Come back in six months," what should you and your parents do? Forget about it? Go to another doctor? Spend the next six months worrying?

The answer to all three questions is "no." First of all, coming back in six months is not forgetting about it. The Scoliosis Association maintains that observation is a form of treatment. You'll most likely feel relieved that you don't have to wear a brace or have surgery, at least for now. On the other hand, the same rules apply for the "wait and see" group and for those who got a clean bill of health: you may have nothing to worry about now, but it never hurts to take care of your body. A good physical fitness regimen will help strengthen your muscles and improve your posture.

If you do need follow-up, there is no need to panic. Your scoliosis was detected before it could get worse. Remember, most people live happy and productive lives with scoliosis. You'll meet some of them in the coming chapters.

On to the Doctor

When she was eleven, Sara-Marie Stefanski visited her doctor for a regular checkup. Her mother mentioned that Sara-Marie sometimes complained of mild back pain after gym class. The doctor took a closer look, performed the Adams Forward-Bend Test, and said that Sara-Marie had a slight case of scoliosis and should see an orthopedist.

Sara-Marie's experience wasn't so different from my own. After my gym teacher alerted her, my mother took me to our family doctor. He ordered an X ray, which showed that I had a marked curvature of the spine. And then he did something for which I will always be grateful: he advised my mother to take me to an orthopedist in New York, 130 miles from my home, who was a specialist in scoliosis. It was quite a distance to travel, but it was worth it to see a doctor who was familiar with scoliosis.

Which Doctor?

Pediatricians are doctors who specialize in the treatment of children and adolescents. They may be the first to notice a problem, often during a routine exam. If someone else, such as a school nurse, teacher, or parent thinks you may have a scoliosis, you will probably be sent to a pediatrician for confirmation. Or you may be sent to an internist, a doctor who specializes in general internal medicine. Some internists are called family practitioners or general practitioners, meaning that they treat both adults and children. If your family routinely uses an internist, check that he or she accepts adolescents as patients, since not all of them do.

Some pediatricians have chosen to specialize in adolescent medicine. If you are uncomfortable about visiting a doctor whose office is swarming with babies and toddlers, and if the family's internist won't see you, ask your parents if you can go to a pediatrician who specializes in treating adolescents. They aren't always easy to find, but a large medical center may be able to refer you to one.

If the doctor—pediatrician, internist, or family practitioner—agrees that you have a problem, he or she will probably refer you to an orthopedist, preferably one who specializes in scoliosis. Orthopedics is the medical specialty concerned with the treatment of the spine, arms and legs, and associated structures. It is fairly easy to find an orthopedist who specializes in spinal deformities. Your pediatrician or general practitioner may either refer you directly or ask a general orthopedist to recommend someone specializing in scoliosis. Also, you or your parents can call the orthopedic department of a large medical center and ask for the name of a scoliosis specialist.

If there is a chapter of the Scoliosis Association, Inc., in your area, this may be the time to look them up. The association is an information and support network with chapters all over the country. It is made up of volunteers, most of whom either have scoliosis themselves or have a family member who does. While the chapter will probably not make specific recommendations, they can give you names of local doctors who specialize in spinal deformities. In addition, they may be able to refer you to chapter members who have consulted those doctors and are willing to discuss their experiences with you.

Another excellent source of information is the Scoliosis Research Society (SRS), an organization of orthopedic surgeons specializing in spinal deformity. The society can give you a list of its members in your geographic area. Physicians cannot join SRS unless at least 20 percent of their practice is devoted to spinal deformity. Doctors who are members of SRS are kept up to date on advances in scoliosis treatment and research by attending SRS meetings. So although the society cannot recommend a specific physician and not every scoliosis specialist belongs to the society, the list is a good place to start.

Both the Scoliosis Association, Inc., and the Scoliosis Research Society are included in the Where to Go for Help section at the end of this book, as is the National Scoliosis Foundation. The foundation, an advocacy organization that publishes informative booklets and tapes about scoliosis, also promotes school screening and scoliosis research.

Chiropractic

Chiropractic, a term meaning "done by hand," is a therapeutic system based on the belief that many diseases are the result of some kind of malfunction of the nerves, especially the nerves in the spine. Chiropractors treat diseases through manipulation of, or use of the hands on, the spinal column and related structures. Two terms frequently used in chiropractic are subluxation, which means a misalignment of the vertebrae, and adjustment, the use of manipulation to apply a thrust that corrects the subluxation. Chiropractors are not the only health care professionals who use manipulation, but they rely on it more heavily than do others.

If you ask most people for a definition of the word *chiropractor,* they might say "back doctor," because a chiropractor is the first person many turn to when they have a problem with their backs. Although chiropractors are addressed as "doctor," they are not physicians (medical doctors). They did not graduate from medical school as physicians must. Chiropractors go to chiropractic school. They do not attain the degree of M.D., or medical doctor. However, chiropractors must be licensed to practice.

Chiropractors have successfully relieved back pain for many people. Often orthopedists refer their patients to chiropractors for the treatment of back pain, and an increasing number of health care plans include chiropractic as a covered service. For those with scoliosis, the question is not whether chiropractic can be helpful for back pain but whether it is an effective treatment for scoliosis.

Some chiropractors believe that early chiropractic intervention, beginning when someone is a young child, can prevent or cure scoliosis. But they do not claim that chiropractic is effective in all cases of scoliosis.

Orthopedists, and even some chiropractors, are skeptical about the ability of chiropractic to affect the progress of scoliosis. Chiropractic manipulation as an effective treatment for scoliosis is still unproven.

A Family Affair

As the time to visit the doctor approaches, you and your parents will need to make plans. Who is going with you to the doctor? Is there any information you need to bring with you to assist the doctor in making a diagnosis and treatment plan? Call the doctor's office a week or two in advance to find out if you should bring anything with you. If possible, it's ideal for you to visit the doctor in the company of one or both of your parents. If you are under the age of eighteen, an adult will need to sign off on any treatment plan the doctor recommends. You may also be grateful for their moral support.

You have the right to express your fears and desires to the doctor, and the more you are able to do this, the better. It may be difficult, as doctors can be intimidating. It will help if, before you and your parents see the orthopedic specialist, you sit down together and have a talk. Express your feelings: Are you upset that you may have to wear a brace and scared that the other kids will tease you? Are you angry that you have to go to the doctor and the other kids in your class don't? Or are you confused and frightened of the unknown?

In addition to talking about feelings, you and your parents can accomplish a number of practical tasks. Prepare yourself to answer questions that the doctor will ask: Did anyone in the family have scoliosis? What about some other back deformity, such as an abnormal kyphosis (humpback) or abnormal lordosis (swayback)? Have you had an illness or accident that could be important in determining the cause? How about a fracture or a high fever? The doctor is going to ask your parents if there were any complications before, during, or after your birth. Write down anything you think may be important. Your pediatrician has probably sent your medical history to the orthopedist, but the more you can discuss your own history, the better. Anything you can add to the doctor's report will make the specialist's job easier.

Write down a list of questions and carry it with you so that you remember to ask them when you see the doctor. Practice asking these questions in advance. When you are speaking with the doctor, write down the answers. Feel free to ask questions about things he or she says that you don't understand.

If anyone else in the family has any questions for the doctor, write them down as well. Although most of the scoliosis specialists I have met are friendly and approachable, visiting a specialist for the first time can be intimidating. Most of them work in large medical centers, so that even finding the doctor's office may be a challenge. They are very busy, and although they should give you all the time you need, it helps if you know what you want to ask. Writing things down will make you and your family feel much more in control of the situation, and it will also help the doctor.

Your parents can reassure you that nothing has been decided yet and that, when the doctor makes his or her diagnosis and recommendation, they will make sure that you get a chance to ask any questions or raise issues that are bothering you. Your parents are there to help you.

I've been saying "your parents" or "your family," but I know that usually only one parent or other adult will be able to come with you. Even if you don't live in a one-parent home, there is a good chance that both parents work, or that someone has to stay home with younger children. If neither parent is able to go, perhaps a close relative can accompany you.

The Examination

The day arrives. You and your mom, dad, or other adult set out for the doctor's office. After you've signed in with the receptionist and waited (a Walkman or a good book can help you pass the time), the doctor will ask to see both you and the adults with you.

Before he or she examines you, the doctor will talk to all of you. Your parents will be asked the questions that you've been preparing for: whether there is any family history of scoliosis, and whether you had any problems at birth or in early childhood that might have interfered with the development of your spine. These questions help the doctor to determine whether you have congenital or infantile scoliosis, or if the spine curves as a result of some neurological or muscular disease—muscular dystrophy or cerebral palsy, for example. Your medical history will also help the doctor rule out any conditions that look like scoliosis but aren't.

Then the doctor will examine you. This examination is going to be much more thorough than the school screening or the pediatrician's exam, so be prepared and just relax. It's worth your time and effort to see a doctor who really knows about scoliosis and can tell you whether you have it and, if so, if you need to do something about it.

Once again, you are going to be asked to strip down to your underwear. (At this point, your parents may be asked to wait outside for a few minutes.) The doctor will do a thorough physical, examining you closely and possibly asking you some questions that can sound pretty personal, maybe even a little embarrassing. If you're a girl, he or she may check to see if you have developed breasts, if there's hair under your arms, and may ask if you've had your first period. He or she may ask you to remove your bra, because the placement of your breasts can indicate rib rotation associated with scoliosis. For boys, the doctor will want to know if your penis and testicles have grown to adult proportions, if you have pubic hair, and if you've started to shave.

What has all this personal information got to do with your back? A lot. For most patients, adolescent idiopathic scoliosis progresses most rapidly during the adolescent growth spurt, the time in early adolescence when your growth rate, especially bone growth, speeds up greatly. This spurt comes earlier for girls than for boys, and it ends earlier, at around age sixteen. Boys don't reach their full growth until age eighteen, and sometimes later. Therefore, it's important for the doctor to know whether the age of puberty has been reached and, if so, how far it has progressed.

As you get nearer to physical maturity, evidenced by the beginning of menstruation in girls and the growth of facial hair in boys, the rate of growth slows down. So does the risk that a spinal curve will progress. That doesn't mean that the risk goes down to zero; curves can progress even after full bone growth is reached. However, the likelihood does go down after you've become an adult. The doctor will need to take an X ray to determine bone maturity.

A thorough orthopedic exam comes next. You will be asked to walk away from the doctor, turn around, and walk back. Then you'll sit on the examining table while the doctor examines your extremities (legs and arms) and tests your reflexes. You'll be hit with a small rubber hammer just below each knee. It doesn't hurt, but it will probably cause your leg to jump involuntarily. The doctor is checking to see that both legs react in the same way. If they don't, you may have a weakness on one side caused by a nerve or muscle problem. That would affect the way you stand or walk, which could in turn cause the spine to curve. That's not scoliosis, but it is something that requires attention.

Now the doctor finally focuses on your back, first examining it visually. The specialist's eye is trained to detect any asymmetry (lack of evenness) between the left and right sides of your body. Small differences that even your family or best friends don't notice, especially when you are fully clothed and moving or sitting, will be more apparent to a scoliosis specialist.

After the doctor has taken a good look, he or she will give you the Adams Forward-Bend Test. You'll probably be asked to bend over one time with your back to the doctor, and once again facing him or her. If you have scoliosis, and the scoliosis is in the upper vertebrae, a rib hump will be more visible when you face the doctor; if it's lower, it will be more easily seen from behind.

The appearance of a rib hump means that the spinal curve has caused the ribs on one side of your body to rotate forward and the ribs on the other side to rotate backward. When they go backward, they protrude. This causes a hump to appear when you bend over. A rib hump can be measured with an instrument called a scoliometer. It is somewhat like the level that carpenters use to see if floors, sills, and other surfaces are even. It is a small, rectangular device with a notch in it that fits over the spine. It contains a narrow, curving, fluid-filled glass tube in which a small ball floats. You bend over, the doctor places the scoliometer on your back, and the ball rolls to the lowest point in the tube, enabling the doctor to measure the angle of rotation.

A scoliometer gives the doctor useful information without any harmful side effects to the patient. However, it is only one tool. It doesn't give even the most skilled scoliosis specialist all the necessary information. Also, it measures only certain kinds of curves. The most common kind of curve is a right thoracic curve (a curve in the upper spine that bends toward the right side), and the scoliometer can be a valuable aid in measuring the angle of rotation of these curves. Curves in the upper spine (thoracic curves) usually produce significant rib rotation too, but lower (lumbar) curves may not. A scoliometer is called a noninvasive tool because it doesn't invade the patient's body with potentially harmful agents such as radiation or dyes.

Another noninvasive technique used by many doctors is moiré topography. It requires the patient to stand in front of a lighted grid that casts a pattern of shadows on

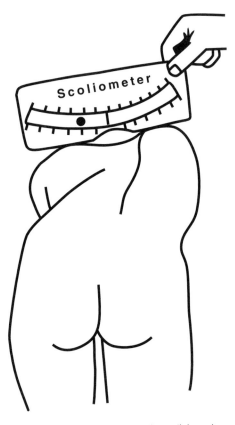

A scoliometer measures how much the ribs have rotated when a rib hump is present.

the patient's back. For scoliosis patients, these shadows look uneven. The patterns are recorded with a Polaroid camera, and the procedure is repeated at each successive visit.

Some doctors and physical therapists use only Polaroid photos of a patient's standing posture, from both the back and the side, to assess the degree to which the curve has progressed. By comparing the pictures, with or without moiré topography, orthopedists can get a fairly clear idea of changes that are taking place over time.

X Rays

If the doctor has diagnosed scoliosis through a physical exam and a scoliometer measurement, he or she will probably order an X ray. X rays give orthopedists information about scoliosis that currently cannot be obtained by any other means. X rays can give doctors a clear picture of the size of the curve, show whether the pelvis is tilted and the hips are not symmetrical, and indicate how mature the spine is.

X rays have proven to be extremely useful in medicine, and the dangers of radiation from exposure to X rays, including increased cancer risk, are well known. That is why X-ray equipment is constantly being improved, as is the knowledge of radiology technicians. It is standard practice for patients to stand at least six feet away from the X-ray machine for a scoliosis X ray. Lead shields are used to protect breasts in girls and penis and testicles in boys. Make sure that the X-ray lab uses lead shields when taking your X rays.

For the initial diagnosis, many orthopedists will have two X rays taken: a front-to-back (called anterior-posterior, or A-P) view, and a wrist X ray to show bone maturity.

Some doctors may ask for a third X ray at this stage, a lateral (sideways) view. This gives information about the sagittal curve of the spine, the gentle S everyone's spine forms as viewed from the side. If, on visual observation, the doctor thinks either of these curves appears too pronounced—abnormal kyphosis (humpback) or abnormal lordosis (swayback)—or not pronounced enough (flat-back), he or she may add the third X ray. However, for an initial diagnosis, it may not be necessary.

How much of the patient do you have to X-ray to get a good look at the spine? A full spinal X ray, about three feet long, should tell doctors everything they need to know. Lead shields must be used to protect sensitive tissue, such as breast tissue and sex organs, from any radiation. If you or your parents have any questions about the safety of the X rays, ask how many X rays are needed and what precautions will be taken, whether the X rays are taken in a large medical center or a freestanding radiology clinic.

If you switch doctors or want to get a second opinion, ask to take the X rays with you or arrange to have them forwarded to the second doctor. The film can be released to you or your family if you have a release form signed by your parent or guardian. There is no need to be X-rayed again if the X-ray films already exist.

Understanding Angles and Scales

Cobb Angles
When doctors or patients talk about scoliosis, they drop numbers like crazy. "He's got a 40-degree right thoracic curve," they may say, or "I have a 50-degree right thoracic curve but only a 30-degree left lumbar curve." What does this mean?

After a spine has been X-rayed, a doctor examines the film. If he or she sees a curve, the doctor will identify the vertebra at the top of the curve (that is, the first vertebra that isn't exactly in line with the one above it). The doctor will draw a horizontal line along the upper edge of that vertebra. The procedure is repeated at the bottom of the curve, with a horizontal line drawn along the lower edge of the bottom vertebra of the curve. Then vertical lines are drawn perpendicular to each horizontal line. The doctors then measure the degree of the angle where the lines meet. This is called the Cobb angle, named after the late Dr. John Cobb of the Hospital for Special Surgery in New York, who developed this system of measuring curves.

Cobb angles are very helpful to orthopedists in establishing one system of classifying curves. A curve of less than 10 degrees is usually considered a "normal deviation." In other words, the spine is supposed to be 100 percent straight, but if it's 95 percent straight, that is also considered normal. A Cobb angle of 20 degrees or less is very mild; 20 to 30 degrees is "wait and see" territory; 30 to 40 degrees is moderate; 40 to 50 degrees is usually the "gray area" between bracing and surgery; and more than 50 degrees is pretty serious.

However, there is some room for interpretation of Cobb angles. Dr. Thomas Haher of St. Vincent's Medical Center, New York, told me that the Scoliosis Research Society gave some spinal X-ray films to a group of scoliosis specialists and asked each to measure the Cobb angles. The results: no two measurements were exactly the same. They weren't dramatically different, but in some instances there was as much as a 5- to 10-degree difference between readings. As a result, Haher prefers to say that a curve is either "mild" or "significant" and not to get hung up on numbers.

At the initial diagnosis stage, the second important

question a doctor will ask in relation to a Cobb angle is, "How much more is this person going to grow?" A curve of 40 degrees in a fifteen-year-old girl or a seventeen-year-old boy is far different from one in an eight-year-old.

Bone Maturity and the Risser Scale

The Risser scale, developed in 1958 by Dr. Joseph Risser, helps physicians determine bone maturity. This scale measures the way the growth plate located on the top of the pelvis matures, changing from cartilage to bone from the outside in. When this bone, which looks like a cap on the top of the pelvis, first appears, doctors know that the patient has about two years of growth remaining. Risser divided the bony cap into four stages, ranging from Risser 1, the most immature, to Risser 4, when the cap is completely formed. When the space between the cap and the pelvis fills in, they call it Risser 5, signifying that full bone growth has been achieved. Of course, the other signs of maturity already described are also considered in evaluating a patient's physical maturity.

The pelvis is visible on the anterior-posterior (A-P) X ray discussed earlier. It shows the spinal curve, so doctors often determine the patient's Risser measurements from one X ray. However, some doctors order an X ray of the hand and wrist, which gives an even clearer picture of skeletal maturity. By analyzing thousands of hand and wrist X rays, doctors have developed standards that allow them to judge the child's or teenager's skeletal (bone) age and estimate how much more the child or teenager will grow. Skeletal age and chronological age are not always the same. A fifteen-year-old may have the bones of a thirteen-year-old or vice versa. The hand and wrist X ray may be ordered at the initial diagnosis or at a later stage, when the doctor is try-ing to decide which treatment is most appropriate.

Putting It Together: The Diagnosis

After the doctor has looked at you and your X rays, he or she is ready to make a diagnosis. If your curve is less than 20 degrees and you are near complete bone maturity, most physicians will not recommend further treatment.

If the curve is more than 20 degrees or you still have a lot of growing to do, the doctor will consider other factors as well. One is the degree of rotation, or how much the vertebrae have turned.

Degree of Rotation

To determine rotation, the doctor will examine your A-P X ray. He or she will draw a vertical line, known as the mid-line, through the middle of each vertebra in the curve.

On the sides of each vertebra are oval indentations, called pedicles, which are visible on the X ray. In a spine that has no rotation, the pedicles are visible on either side of each vertebra, just as most people's two eyes are visible when they face forward. When a person rotates his head in one direction, the position of the eyes also shifts, so that one stays forward but moves sideways, and the other rotates toward the back; when the head is in profile, only one eye is visible. In the spine, when rotation of a verte-bra has occurred, one pedicle stays forward but moves sideways and one rotates farther back.

On the A-P X ray, the pedicles of rotated vertebrae will appear closer to the midline drawn by the doctor than will

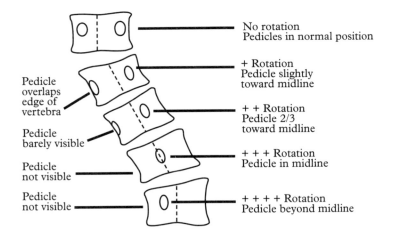

No rotation
Pedicles in normal position

+ Rotation
Pedicle slightly
toward midline

+ + Rotation
Pedicle 2/3
toward midline

+ + + Rotation
Pedicle in midline

+ + + + Rotation
Pedicle beyond midline

Pedicle
overlaps
edge of
vertebra

Pedicle
barely visible

Pedicle
not visible

Pedicle
not visible

When vertebrae have not rotated, both pedicles will be visible in an X ray when the spine is viewed straight on. If rotation has occurred, the position of the pedicles will change according to the amount of rotation of the vertebrae.

the pedicles of unrotated vertebrae. Doctors use numbers to describe the relation of the pedicle to the midline. The closer the pedicle is to the midline, the higher the number; +1 indicates a slight amount of rotation, and +4 a severe amount.

Pain

Finally, pain is a factor in the diagnosis. Most teenagers with idiopathic scoliosis don't have much pain. If they do, however, then some kind of treatment is needed for the pain, even if the curve is relatively small. If they don't have pain, the type of curve and its possibility of causing pain in the future will be taken into consideration.

Hearing the Diagnosis

Listening to the diagnosis is a family affair. The doctor may want to talk to your parents first, or he or she may speak to all of you at the same time. If you don't understand something, make sure you ask questions of both the doctor and your parents.

The doctor will explain the results of the examination—the severity and location of the curve, the degree of rotation, if any, and your skeletal maturity. If the curve is more than 20 degrees and you have a significant amount of growing to do, some treatment will usually be recommended. This treatment may take the form of watchful waiting. But if the curve is more than 30 degrees or if there are any complicating conditions, the doctor may suggest a brace; or, in the most severe cases (usually more than 50 degrees), surgery.

Note that I use words like "recommend" and "suggest." As Dr. Michael Neuwirth, coauthor of *The Scoliosis Handbook,* observes, scoliosis is not an emergency. It is not like pneumonia or appendicitis, where a delay in treatment could be fatal. You and your parents can take your time, ask questions, and then go home and decide on a game plan.

Only two forms of treatment have been scientifically proved to alter the course of scoliosis: bracing, which can stop a curve from getting worse, and surgery, which can correct a curve. Both have advantages and disadvantages. If you choose one, you have to commit yourself to following through. A brace won't help you if it's in the closet. Surgery won't be effective if you don't follow the doctor's orders. But you won't be alone. This is a team effort. Your parents, your doctor, health-care experts, teachers, scoliosis support groups, and close friends can help.

The first thing to do is consider the options, weigh the possible consequences of various courses of action, and make an informed decision. Depending on your spine, you have several options: you can do nothing; adopt a "wait-and-see" attitude; get a brace; or have surgery performed (if a brace doesn't work). Whether or not the orthopedist has recommended bracing or surgery, everyone benefits from knowing good health habits. Even if the orthopedist concluded that you don't have scoliosis or your scoliosis isn't severe, he or she can suggest how you can keep your back healthy.

In the next chapters, we will look at some strategies that help promote good back health. Proper nutrition, exercise, and a positive attitude are good for everyone. By choosing to participate in your own physical development, you will be developing good health habits that will last a lifetime.

Staying Fit Is Good for You

I discovered healthy eating and exercise long after I became an adult. As a result, I feel better now than I did when I was younger. All people, whether or not they have a spinal problem, can benefit from eating and exercising right. There are also physical therapy and fitness regimens that are specifically geared for scoliosis and kyphosis patients.

Milk Does Your Body Good

I'm sure you know something about what you should and shouldn't eat. Your parents have probably been on your case about eating fresh fruits and vegetables and drinking plenty of milk, and you've probably also studied the five basic food groups, or their successor, the Food and Drug Administration's food pyramid, in school. Even advertisements insist that it's cool to drink milk. Most kids have been told that they should eat and drink the right foods, but do they?

Students in three Long Island, New York, schools and one Brooklyn school were asked to keep track of everything they ate for a week, in order to see how close they came to the daily quota of five fruits and vegetables recommended by the National Cancer Institute. Each of the eighty-seven children polled averaged slightly less than five servings of fruits and vegetables a week, with only one student eating anywhere near the ideal—a little over three servings a day. That's after the researchers subtracted french fries—not exactly what nutritionists have in mind under the category of vegetables.

Sound familiar? If it's been a while since you settled down to watch TV with a bag of carrot sticks by your side, or if you prefer soda to milk as your lunch and dinner beverage, don't relax and say, "Everybody's doing it." The rules weren't formulated to make your life miserable. They are based on many years of documented research. If you break the rules, you're only cheating yourself.

Childhood and adolescence are the periods when that intricate structure called the human body is being built. Just as a building is only as good as the bricks, wood, and steel that go into it, your body won't function right without the correct building blocks.

Proper nutrition, essential to growth, means consuming a wide variety of foods. You need proteins, carbohydrates, vitamins, minerals, and yes, even fats (though not too many or the wrong kind) all your life, but especially during the adolescent growth spurt. If you get too little nutrition, your growth, both physical and mental, can be impaired. Anorexia and bulimia are serious health problems for teens and should be treated immediately. On the other hand, if you eat too much of the wrong kind of food and don't exercise enough, you can become overweight. Being overweight can exert a strain on your back and cause other health problems. Both extremes must be avoided.

Let's concentrate on the nutritional elements that most

directly affect the development of the musculoskeletal system, of which your spine is a major part. There is little or no evidence that improper nutrition causes scoliosis. But we do know that certain elements contained in food help strong bones and muscles grow, and that most of that growth takes place during your teens. If your bones and muscles are not strong, any spinal problems you do have can get worse.

Calcium is important for your body. You need calcium to help bones and muscles grow and develop. It can also help prevent osteoporosis, or brittle bones, which can affect people as they get older. However, the stronger your bones become now, the less worry you will have in the future.

Milk and milk products (cheese, cottage cheese, yogurt) give you protein and calcium for strong bones, teeth, and muscles. If you haven't achieved your full bone growth yet (which occurs at around age sixteen for girls and eighteen for boys), you'll need four servings a day. After you reach maturity, you may need fewer servings, but calcium is still important. If you need to keep fat consumption down, remember that skim and low-fat milk products are just as good a source of protein and calcium as whole milk. If you are still growing and exercise a lot, your body does need some fat, but use good judgment. Eating a lot of high-fat, high-sugar ice cream, for example, may spoil your appetite for other, healthful foods, and lead to bad health habits.

Calcium is a mineral, one of a group called "macrominerals"—which means that the body needs large quantities of them, as opposed to "trace" minerals, of which a much smaller quantity is required. Vitamin D helps the body absorb calcium, and it too is contained in milk and milk products. You can also get vitamin D from tuna fish and eggs. The sun is an excellent source of vitamin D, but there is a real risk of skin cancer from overexposure to sunlight. It's fine to be outdoors in the summer if you remember to use a good sunscreen. However, sunbathing for hours can damage your skin, even with sunscreen.

It's a common error to think milk and dairy products are the only way you can get calcium. Fish and shellfish are also an excellent source. Three ounces of sardines canned in oil yield 372 milligrams of calcium, more than an eight-ounce glass of milk. Green vegetables like broccoli, collard greens, and turnip greens are also rich in calcium.

The simplest way to make sure you get enough calcium and vitamin D is to drink four eight-ounce glasses of milk a day. Or drink three glasses—one with each meal—and get the fourth serving from other dairy products, seafood, or green vegetables. Unfortunately, kids don't drink as much milk as their bodies need. The survey of children in four New York-area schools mentioned earlier found that they were more likely to drink soda with a meal, or possibly even coffee or tea. By doing this they are cheating their bodies of an essential mineral.

If you really hate the taste of milk, then try flavoring it with a couple of teaspoons of chocolate powder or a shot of chocolate syrup. A half-teaspoon of vanilla and a teaspoon of sugar in milk also tastes good. The sugar isn't the greatest thing in the world for you, but it's a lot better than not drinking milk. On cold days, a cup of hot chocolate is nice, and you can make it with skim or low-fat milk if the extra calories are a problem.

Some people can't drink milk, or think they can't. Some

babies and children are allergic to cow's milk. Milk substitutes, usually soybean-based, are prescribed for them. Soybeans are another important source of calcium. One three-and-one-half-ounce serving of tofu (bean curd) provides 130 milligrams of calcium, nearly as much as one-half cup of pudding made with skim milk. Soy milk, too, has calcium.

Recently, a condition called lactose intolerance (an inability to digest lactose, the complex sugar contained in milk) has received a lot of publicity. However, research shows that a lot of people who think they are lactose intolerant really aren't. Either their symptoms come from some other condition, or they simply drink too much milk too fast or on an empty stomach. Often, when they drink smaller quantities of milk and drink milk with meals, their symptoms disappear. For people who are really lactose intolerant, reduced-lactose milk and tablets that aid in the digestion of lactose are sold in most supermarkets. Also, not all milk products contain the same amount of lactose. Buttermilk, some yogurts, and many cheese products have very little lactose.

Bones need not only calcium but also protein, which is essential for strong muscles and healthy blood. Meats, poultry, fish, eggs, dried beans, and peas are all protein sources. Have two or three servings a day.

What about fats? A little bit of fat goes a long way. A small serving of fat (about a teaspoon of margarine, butter, mayonnaise or oil; a tablespoon of salad dressing; an ounce of nuts; or a slice of bacon) three times a day is as much as you need. Fats provide fatty acids, calories, and vitamins A, D, and E for growth.

Vitamins are important to everyone's diet. That doesn't mean that all you have to do is take some vitamin pills and then eat whatever you want. Vitamins come from food, and most people can get all they need by eating the right foods. As for fast food, less is better than more. Double cheeseburgers do have protein (beef and cheese) and calcium (cheese), but they also have loads of animal fat. As for the french fries, potatoes are vegetables that are a great source of carbohydrates and vitamins, but the deep frying in oil makes them a poor food choice.

Not all fast foods are equally bad. A vegetarian pizza is fine, and more and more fast-food places are broiling the burgers instead of frying them. Grilled instead of fried chicken sandwiches are also available. And while you're at the restaurant, be sure to check out the salad bar and build yourself a tossed salad with lettuce, tomatoes, carrots, crunchy vegetables, and a little light dressing. Avoid macaroni and potato salad. Just because something is on the salad bar doesn't mean it's good for you.

Smoking and Alcohol

While there are no data linking smoking and alcohol consumption directly to scoliosis, both of these lifestyle choices pose a serious health hazard to teens. They are even more of a risk for young people with scoliosis and related spinal irregularities.

Researchers believe that at least 40 percent of young people seventeen or under smoke or used to smoke, although only 26 percent admit to being smokers. We do know that 71 percent of people who have ever smoked cigarettes started before they were eighteen, and that 90 percent of beginning smokers are children and teens. Every day, more than 3,000 U.S. teens light up for the first time. If current trends hold true, one-third of these will die someday of diseases related to tobacco consumption.

Smoking has been proven to affect the heart and lungs, causing emphysema, lung cancer, and heart disease. Because severe scoliosis can also interfere with maximum heart and lung efficiency, smoking may pose an additional risk for someone with scoliosis.

For anyone undergoing surgery for scoliosis, there is an even more compelling reason not to smoke. Researchers from the University of Texas Southwestern Medical School found that smokers' broken bones took 276 days to heal, as compared with 146 for nonsmokers—almost twice as long. They think this is because smoking interferes with blood circulation to the bone. What does this have to do with scoliosis? While only a fraction of people with scoliosis ever have surgery, this finding could mean that a scoliosis patient who smokes will recover much more slowly from surgery than a nonsmoker.

Although it is illegal for those under twenty-one to buy or consume alcoholic beverages, many teenagers do drink—to feel cool, to deal with shyness, or because their friends do it. But for teens at risk for scoliosis, it should be noted that long-term heavy use of alcohol can cause loss of appetite and vitamin deficiency, robbing your body of essential nutrients necessary for bone growth and development.

Smoking and drinking don't cause scoliosis, but they do interfere with overall health and the development of good health habits. And the healthier your body, especially your bones and muscles, the more easily you will be able to deal with scoliosis if it develops.

Building a Better You

Being physically fit and engaging in sports can be two entirely different things. If you play sports or work out only every once in a while, chances are that you're not staying physically fit. Physical fitness requires regular exercise. Of course, athletes who want to succeed have to stay in shape, and lots of sports, especially noncontact sports such as swimming, help you to stay in shape. But for teens, staying fit helps develop a healthy body and a good self-image, especially during the years of maximum growth. This is a good goal in itself.

If you wear a brace, or if you will soon have or have recently had surgery, it is important to follow your doctor's recommendations about sports and exercise. Doing so will allow you to achieve maximum benefit from your therapy.

For those with milder cases of scoliosis, check with your doctor concerning what sports and exercises will be especially beneficial or should be avoided, if any. For most of you, the following discussion is relevant—but always check with your doctor before engaging in any of these activities. Like the rest of this book, this information is provided to assist you in understanding and living with scoliosis, and is not intended to be a substitute for informed medical opinion.

Exercise!

During adolescence, it's important to be physically active. Competitive sports are fine, but the main person to compete with is yourself. A regular physical fitness program develops bones, muscles, and organs, such as your heart and lungs. Furthermore, by sticking to a routine, you learn self-discipline. By developing your skills in a sport, you can build self-confidence and self-esteem. You can also feel a sense of accomplishment through working toward a personal goal and achieving it. Participating in a sport can be a good way to establish and accomplish some goals.

Exercise comes in two general categories: aerobic and anaerobic. Aerobic activities increase your heart rate while you are doing them. They develop muscle flexibility and heart and lung capacity. Anaerobic activities are marked by short bursts of intense effort followed by periods of rest; some examples are weight lifting, sit-ups, and push-ups. Anaerobic exercises increase muscle strength.

Aerobic activities are very important during adolescence, especially during the growth spurt. The best-known aerobic activities are running, walking (briskly), and swimming. Some others are bicycling, cross-country skiing, ice skating, karate, and rowing. Some anaerobic activities, such as sit-ups and weight lifting, can be harmful for people with certain kinds of back problems.

To be aerobic, exercise must be maintained for at least twenty minutes at a stretch. To have any lasting benefit, it has to be done at least three times a week. It's better to do some exercise every week than a big burst one week and nothing the next. That just confuses your body and does not help anyone. Ideally, exercise such as swimming or bicycle riding should be in addition to the exercises you do at home to stretch your muscles.

Try to do some kind of muscle stretches every day. Maybe you'd like to practice some of the exercises you do in gym class, or ask your gym teacher to show you some simple stretches you can do at home. You may want to check local television listings and find a fitness program that's on while you are at home. If it's on when you're not home, you might be able to videotape it. There are also a lot of workouts on video. Go to the local video store or public library and check out a few so that you can select one that's right for you. That way you can select fifteen or twenty minutes' worth of stretches, learn them, and do them every day.

It's not true that if some aerobic exercise is good, more is better and even more is even better than that. Avoid overdoing it. Save some strength for the next time. If you don't have enough breath left to sing while you're biking or running, but you are still able to talk, then your pace is just about right.

Alternative Therapies

So far, we've been talking about sports and exercises that everyone is familiar with. No one would argue with the fact that walking or swimming is good for you. But other programs have been suggested for improving physical fitness and alleviating back pain that aren't as well known but are gaining in popularity. Adolescence, a time of growth and change, is a good time to learn new ways of moving and thinking about your body. For people with postural scoliosis, or mild structural scoliosis or kyphosis—as well as those with scoliosis whose only treatment is "wait and see"—these programs are worth trying. Some may also be used as a physical fitness program for people whose scoliosis does require medical treatment, though not as a substitute for treatment.

What are these other approaches, known as alternative therapies? They include yoga, the Feldenkrais Method, the Pilates Method, and more. These and other alternative therapies are sometimes called "alternative medicine," "bodywork," or "movement therapy." One thing to keep in mind is that none of these techniques has been tested using scientific methods, and they have not been proven through scientific research to correct scoliosis. Only bracing and surgery have been scientifically proven to be effective in stopping or correcting a spinal curvature. However, some people with scoliosis have found that these alternative therapies give them a sense of physical and emotional well-being, as well as stretching and strengthening muscles and enhancing their overall health.

By teaching you to be aware of your body, bodywork and yoga can improve your balance, posture and self-image. They can boost your self-confidence and help you move more easily and even have less back pain.

There are a few rules of thumb that might help you to decide if you want to explore these alternatives. They include:

1. **Cost-effectiveness:** If it costs too much—either in time or money—don't do it. Your money and your time are limited, so the system has to be worth the expense and effort. None of these systems is free. You have to learn each from a teacher. There may

be some videos available, but I wouldn't recommend them except as supplements to formal instruction. Often you have to use special equipment or machines that are available only in a gym or studio. It may be worth checking with your health insurance provider to see if the cost of particular alternative therapies is covered. Some insurers do cover them, particularly when they have been prescribed by a doctor.

2. **Active participation with support:** An alternative therapy that teaches you something—such as a new awareness of your body and its movements; a new way to stand, sit, and walk; or exercises you can do at home—is especially valuable. Active participation gives you a measure of control: you're doing the exercise, so you can tell if something doesn't feel right and can stop before you injure yourself. At the same time, it's good to have support, in the form of either a piece of equipment or a teacher who holds you steady and guides your movements. Support helps you learn and prevents injury.

3. **Trust and chemistry:** You've got to have a teacher you trust and who is right for you. The first step is to find someone who comes well recommended. Next the person must be someone you like and respect, someone from whom you're willing to accept constructive criticism and who will listen to your questions and comments.

Bodywork and Movement Techniques

Three bodywork systems are the Alexander Technique, the Feldenkrais Method, and the Pilates Method. The Alexander Technique, one of the oldest and best known of these methods, is not used as much in connection with problems associated with scoliosis as are Feldenkrais and Pilates. But the ideas behind the Alexander Technique have influenced the development of other bodywork systems.

Alexander Technique

Frederick Matthias Alexander observed that habits of faulty posture—as in sitting and standing—contribute to physical and emotional problems. He developed a method by which to rebalance the body. The Alexander Technique is intended to make a person become aware of unhealthy movements and postures, learn how to interrupt ineffective habits of posture and movement, and practice new ways of thinking about and moving the body. The aim is to restore good use of the body, particularly by improving the relationship between the head, the neck, and the back.

Students of the Alexander Technique learn how to improve their motion, balance, and posture. One of the direct descendants of the Alexander Technique is the Feldenkrais Method.

Feldenkrais Method

Moshe Feldenkrais was a Russian-born Israeli physicist. When an old soccer-related knee injury of his flared up, he began an in-depth study of human movement and its relation to behavior. By teaching himself how to use his knee correctly, he alleviated his pain. This led him to develop the Feldenkrais Method, which is now taught by practitioners throughout the world.

Mary Newell was in her twenties when she began to experience back pain. "Living in California, I had tried just about everything," she said. She finally turned to Feldenkrais and found that it helped her "so much that I wanted to use it to help other people." Newell is now a certified Feldenkrais practitioner.

"Feldenkrais deals with function, not just structure," Newell told me in an interview. "A Feldenkrais practitioner will look at what you can and can't do well and will analyze it from a dynamic [movement] perspective." Newell would like to have more opportunity to work with teenagers, especially those with mild scoliosis whose curves have not yet progressed. "One of the problems in working with younger people with scoliosis," she says, "is that often they don't know they have it until someone tells them."

Feldenkrais is taught in group classes, called Awareness Through Movement, or in private Functional Integration sessions. Students usually work lying on the floor or on a table, to counteract the pull of gravity on the body. In Awareness Through Movement classes, students work through a series of movements and exercises, being careful to stay within their comfort range and not to reach the point of pain. "The participants are guided through a graduated series of movements," says Newell of the classes. One-on-one private sessions with an instructor are also available. Here, Newell says, "individuals are helped to improve a functional difficulty or, for instance, to perfect technique in sports or music. The gentle and nonintrusive hands-on work allows a letting go of deep-seated contractions that contribute to pain."

I asked Newell how she adapts this method to working with scoliosis patients, and she replied: "One of the approaches of Feldenkrais is that you kind of take over the work of the body. If someone has a curvature to the right and a rotation to the left, I would actually support the person in that and, if it's not too extreme, I might go a little more in that direction. Then the brain, which is holding that pattern, would give up all that extra work and stop holding it. This is sometimes extremely effective, particularly in earlier cases where the vertebrae haven't yet become malformed. Very often there's a lot of muscular holding, which the person doesn't know she is doing. The brain has just been set to do this. When I take over all that work, the brain says, 'Ahh,' and it sends in a whole different set of signals. After that, sometimes you find that the person can move in the other direction much more; there's much more possibility."

For more information on the Feldenkrais Method or for the name of a Feldenkrais practitioner in your area, you can write the Feldenkrais Guild, listed in the Where to Go for Help section. Feldenkrais will not correct structural scoliosis, but it can help people move better and develop a better self-image. Moshe Feldenkrais called himself a teacher, not a therapist, and his system is a way of reeducating the body to achieve better balance and movement.

Pilates Method

Pilates is certainly not new, but it's enjoying new popularity. Its founder, Joseph Pilates, a German born in 1880, was a sickly child who learned how to overcome his illnesses by studying anatomy, physiology, exercise, and physical therapy. In the 1920s he established the American Foundation for Physical Fitness in New York. Pilates's exercises were aimed at developing muscle power while increasing body awareness and flexibility.

Sean P. Gallagher is a physical therapist who heads the Pilates Studio® in New York. For five years, he was a physical therapist for the New York City Ballet. Athletes and dancers often use the Pilates technique to tone up or as part of their physical therapy regimen when recovering from injuries.

When I visited the studio to interview Gallagher I got a real treat—a half-hour session with a teacher familiar with scoliosis. Unfortunately, it's impossible to describe the session in detail. What I do remember about the session was that I came out of it with a feeling of well-being and a healthy respect for the skill of my instructor.

"The Alexander Technique, Feldenkrais, and Pilates all focus on body awareness and neuromuscular reeducation," Sean Gallagher explained to me. "However, the Alexander Technique focuses on the head and neck, while for both Feldenkrais and Pilates the pelvis area is central. Feldenkrais stresses mobility, Pilates stability." To Joseph Pilates, the abdomen, lower back, and buttocks are the center of the body's power, making it possible for the rest of the body to move freely.

In addition, "Pilates differs from Feldenkrais because it

uses resistance," Gallagher told me. "All our equipment has springs, which can be adjusted to the needs of the student."

One piece of equipment used in Pilates is called a Reformer. The Reformer is a platform with a padded bench-type bed. You can perform exercises in a standing, sitting, kneeling, or lying position. The bed is moved during the exercises by pulling on straps with your arms or with your legs by pushing on a bar. Other equipment is also used. Some Pilates exercises don't require a lot of specialized equipment, although it's not a good idea to try to do them without first having a Pilates instructor show you how. These exercises are done on a mat on the floor and at first glance look like some of the sit-ups, leg lifts, and other exercises you may be familiar with. However, the mat exercises, like those done on the Reformer, are unique to Pilates.

All Pilates exercises aim at developing the body's "powerhouse"—the abdomen, back, and buttocks. Joseph Pilates reasoned that if the body's core is stable, it takes pressure off the arms and legs and improves breathing, balance, and posture. Pilates can help people with mild scoliosis or with postural problems that can be mistaken for scoliosis.

Balance is important to Pilates. One of the purposes of the Reformer and other equipment is to set boundaries and center the body. Arms and legs can't stray off to one side when one is lying on the narrow table of the Reformer or standing within the Tower, a vertical frame that looks like a doorway with adjustable springs attached.

"The Pilates method can compensate for a body that's been unevenly developed by athletics," says Gallagher.

But you don't have to wait until damage has been done. Pilates is a great workout for everybody.

You can order some of the Pilates equipment for home use, but it is relatively costly, and you definitely shouldn't use it unless you have been instructed by a certified Pilates trainer. The alternative is to take lessons at a studio until you progress to the point at which you can come in and use the equipment unsupervised. Either way requires a commitment of time and money, but if you are willing and able to make this commitment, you may want to explore this bodywork system further.

If you're interested in learning more about Pilates, you can write the Pilates Studio® in New York (see Where to Go for Help) for a list of certified studios or instructors near you. Also, Pilates has a site on the World Wide Web, where you can read more about the method.

Yoga

Yoga is an ancient system of exercises that strives to achieve physical and mental control and well-being. Yoga will not cure scoliosis, but it can help strengthen your mind and body and reduce stress.

Bobbie Fultz developed scoliosis around age eleven. When she was in her teens, she saw Richard Hittleman and his assistant, Diana, demonstrating hatha yoga on television. "I was very impressed by Diana because of her grace and her expression of serenity," says Fultz. Fultz explored a number of options to relieve her back pain and internal complications related to her curvature. But it was that early experience that influenced her to devote her life to the study and teaching of yoga.

Today she teaches the style of yoga developed by the Indian guru B. K. S. Iyengar. Iyengar yoga uses props—pillows, blankets, belts, mats—to support and align the body and thus prevent injury. Although it can be beneficial to anyone, Iyengar yoga is especially suitable for people with scoliosis and other spinal problems.

Yoga has helped Fultz cope with her own scoliosis. She uses the word "collapse" to describe the effects of scoliosis on the body. It's easy to understand why: Instead of expanding upward, the spine curves downward on one side, compressing the structures on that side. Fultz's own history gives a dramatic example of this.

"The progression of the collapse of my spine," she says, "was most noticeable to me by my gradual loss of height. Each year that I was measured during physical exams I was told that I was shorter than the previous year. I measured five feet eight and one-half inches at age eighteen. I already had a significant collapse, so I probably never reached my full height potential. By the time I was thirty-five, I stood less than five feet six inches. As I began my intense yoga practice, I used this yardstick to measure my progress. I regained one-half inch in the first two years; one-half inch during my first study in India with Mr. Iyengar; and another one-half inch the year after that experience, when I was inspired to work at home every day. I no longer measure my height. Now I can measure my progress by my mobility in different yoga poses and which poses my body is now capable of performing.

"Yoga is a holistic practice of well-being," Fultz says. "The idea is that the body desires to be healthy, and if we give it the direction and the support that it needs, it will strive toward health and balance. One of the biggest misconceptions about yoga is that you need to be flexible or strong to come into yoga. If we had to wait for that, there would be no yoga classes."

Proper stretching and breathing—recommended in almost all physical fitness programs—are central to yoga. The first pose Fultz teaches involves nothing more than standing straight against a wall, with feet together, shoulders back, and eyes looking straight ahead. She insists that students fan their toes as wide apart as possible, while keeping their heels and big toes touching. To compensate for imbalances in posture, she tells students to take cues from the environment around them. "Level your eyes," she says. This means finding a point directly ahead of you and consciously keeping your head straight as you look at it.

This posture—called *tadasana*, or "mountain posture"—is the basis for most of the other poses, which help stretch the arms and legs while keeping the body centered. Then there is the upside-down work, using ropes, belts, pillows, and other props. "At the end of the day, when gravity's been hauling on you and your own body weight has been leaning on the discs between your vertebrae, everybody's discs compress, and those with scoliosis even more so," Fultz explains.

Some of the postures most identified with hatha yoga, such as standing on the head, can be too heavy for those with a lot of misalignment in the neck or upper back from scoliosis. Iyengar yoga offers a variety of ways to support the body's weight with props to make these actions safe and beneficial. A trained teacher can guide people with scoliosis, especially those who have had surgery, for their specific needs.

"One of the things that's so intriguing about bodywork—all the different systems, whether it's Alexander or Feldenkrais," says Fultz, "is that the significance of holding patterns in the body and releasing is regarded in the same manner. When you are sad or angry, you tighten. When you release, old memories, tastes, and smells come back. There are many different ways of getting to the same result."

Yoga, like Feldenkrais and Pilates, requires a commitment of time and money. If there is an Iyengar studio near you, you might want to take an introductory class before making any decisions. If you have scoliosis and there's a yoga and scoliosis workshop, that's even better.

"One of the reasons I really admire Mr. Iyengar is that he doesn't make it hard on people," says Fultz. "The only commitment you have to make is to begin. Start taking a class once a week. As you come to enjoy the yoga, it becomes part of your life. Your body desires this activity. You become accustomed to taking class for an hour or hour and a half. As in studying any topic, you begin to do the activity at home. You can start a home practice of fifteen minutes. Soon you progress to a practice as long as the classes you are accustomed to attending."

Bodywork is helpful, especially if, in addition to making you feel better physically, it makes you feel better about yourself and improves your self-image.

Building a Strong Self-Image

Michelle Ann Mauney was Miss North Carolina 1995. She is everything you would imagine a beauty queen to be: beautiful, talented, poised, and in great physical shape. There's just one small thing "wrong" with Michelle: a neck-to-tailbone scar down her back, a souvenir of her scoliosis surgery. Even after the surgery, Michelle still has scoliosis, but she carries herself so confidently that most people never notice.

Today Michelle travels around the country giving motivational talks to teenagers, those with scoliosis and those without. She speaks about overcoming adversity, a subject on which she is an authority. In addition to the scoliosis surgery, she had heart surgery when she was four years old, to correct a birth defect.

When I was eighteen, I attended a summer religious study program. There were about twenty-five of us, college students and counselors. The first night, we all had to tell the others a little bit about ourselves—where we came from, what we did, and what some of our most important experiences were. Two people began with, "There has not been one day in my life that I would consider entirely unhappy or wasted." They were a man who, as a child, had

72

escaped from Nazi Germany just before the Holocaust and a woman who, as a teen soldier, had fought in a war. No one else in a room full of comfortable, middle-class Americans felt equally inspired to make that statement.

Ever since that day, I have believed that being happy or sad, a success or a failure, is nine-tenths how you see yourself. Neither of those two people had lived a carefree, pampered youth. Yet both had taken something positive out of every day of their existence. Because how we see ourselves is so important, it is worthwhile to discuss self-image before considering the issues of scoliosis treatment.

Learning you have scoliosis can be traumatic, especially during adolescence. You have a right to feel upset, even angry. But after that, it's important to move on. Michelle's life hasn't been easy, but she has accepted each problem as a challenge. She's also had a lot of support—from her parents, her doctor, and other people with scoliosis. You don't have to face scoliosis alone. There are plenty of places to get help. You just have to know how to ask for it.

Asking for Help

I attended a college that had a peculiar system of assigning rooms to students. Freshman rooms and roommates were assigned with the clear understanding that this was a one-year deal. At the end of the year, there was a lottery. The people with the lowest numbers could pick any room they wanted. The higher your number, the more limited your choice. The only hope for those with high numbers was to have a friend with a low number. By "averaging out," they had a chance of getting a desirable room.

My number was 300—very high. However, I had three or four friends, some of whom had really low numbers. If one of them would room with me, we could share a double room in the dormitory of our choice. I was shy, so I didn't march up to anyone and ask if I could room with her. I just announced my number and waited hopefully. One day, I was in a stall in the bathroom when two girls came in, one a member of my "group." They began to discuss lottery numbers, and the girl who was not a member of our group asked the other girl if she would be inviting me to room with them. "Oh, no," said my "friend." "She wouldn't fit in."

I waited in the stall, too embarrassed to come out. When I did, I managed to control myself through dinner and then went to the library, found a secluded table, and burst into tears. An acquaintance—we'll call her Jane— came in, saw me crying, and asked what the matter was. After she had heard my story, she said, "Did you ever watch a big kettle of water come to a boil? First there are just a few bubbles, then a few more. Finally, the whole pot is bubbling.

"People are like that. As kids, we seem more or less alike, just one big pot of water. Then one or two individuals pop to the surface, then more, and finally everyone has developed a unique personality. That girl didn't know it, but she paid you a compliment by saying you don't fit in. You don't. You are one of the people who bubbled first. You're a distinct individual; you can't be easily pigeonholed. That can be painful now, but it will be fine later on." She suggested that I take a single room in the dormitory where she was going to live. I did, and it turned out to be the perfect place for me.

Telling this story brings back painful memories. I thought at the time that I was the most insecure teenager on earth. I've found out since that Jane was right. All teens are in the process of "bubbling," and while the process is taking place—when the kettle has first been placed on the stove—they take comfort in trying to be like everyone else. They want to wear the same clothes, engage in the same sports, practically think the same thoughts. But there's something you didn't know about your friends and classmates. They really aren't all the same—they only seem that way. As hard as everyone may try to fit in and be the same, we're all different.

I learned two things from my experience with Jane: One was that, even though your "friends" aren't always trustworthy, friendship and help can come from unlikely places. I also learned that Jane was right. People who mature earlier, who stand out from the crowd, may not have an easy time when they are teens, but they usually become successful, happy adults.

The Big Picture

Carla and John Podzius are a husband and wife who help teens and families cope with scoliosis. Carla, a certified social worker with scoliosis, is executive director of the Scoliosis Association of Westchester, New York. She wore a brace in her teens and had a spinal fusion as an adult, so she knows the problems scoliosis can bring from personal experience. John is a psychologist.

Carla and John agree that scoliosis is a problem for teens—an additional hurdle to be overcome at a time when life seems full of hurdles. Yet it is a hurdle that can be overcome. The Podziuses believe that the way you view yourself is the key to dealing with scoliosis successfully.

"I know of some [teenage girls who wear braces] and, especially with the baggy clothes they wear today, you can hardly notice the braces," Carla said. "One might look like a normal kid and act like a normal kid. You would never know she had a brace. Then you have another girl; it's just the same—you can't see the brace. Your perception is just that she's a beautiful teenage girl; she's very pretty. But her perception is that she's ugly and she's defective, she's abnormal. And it's coloring not only her psyche, but her physical look as well. She's a pretty girl, but her face—she's constricting herself; she's avoiding social activity; she has this perception of herself.

"What we're working on always is the perception, not the reality. Reality is the same for all the kids—they're all a certain age, they're teenagers, and they're wearing braces. It's the perception they have that's going to make it or break it."

Self-perception, John says, can be used to positive advantage. "The teen with scoliosis must perceive herself as making a *real* difference in her own health and well-being." John urges teens to be an active part of their program plan and treatment team. This team should include the teen, her physician, and her family. "Of course, she must also be praised for her effort, compliance and accomplishment—for her daily hard work over weeks, months, and years. In this sense, self-perception can make all the difference."

Carla believes a negative self-image can be overcome with help. She thinks it is important to ask others for help, such as your parents, teachers, or friends. People who are close to you can assist you in looking at the bigger picture and help you to realize your strengths as well as interests you may have had in the past, activities you enjoy now, and things you may want to do in the future. They can also help identify times, no matter how brief, when scoliosis has not been a factor in your daily life. Carla believes focusing on these issues can help you come to the realization that, "Yes, all right, I have a brace, but do you know what? I'm great in math, and I have an idea that I may have a career in something interesting to me, and I have a family, and I'm involved in these activities." Scoliosis doesn't have to define your life.

You may feel different from the person next to you because you have scoliosis, but she may be self-conscious about her hair color, her flat feet, or her grade-point average. Realizing that you are different is part of growing up. If you look at scoliosis as a challenge and a learning experience, it can be a giant step toward maturity. This kind of attitude can make you feel much better about yourself and allow you to accomplish more in life.

It's one thing to say, "Develop a positive self-image," but it's another thing to do it. While everybody's situation is different, two general rules may help. First, look at the big picture, and, second, don't try to go it alone.

As Carla says, scoliosis is only part of your life—a very small part, really. It's important to put it in perspective. You are still the same person the day after a diagnosis of scoliosis as you were before. You have the same family and interests, go to the same school, and hang out with the same friends.

However, you may find as time goes on that scoliosis does change certain aspects of your life—sometimes for the better.

"In a way scoliosis created a balance in my life," says Carla Podzius. "I was very sports-minded when I was young. That's where I got all my kudos from my teachers and my brothers." When Carla was diagnosed with scoliosis and began wearing a brace, she started to hang around with the class "brain," and in eighth grade they became best friends. This new friend helped Carla realize there was a lot to life beyond sports.

"What scoliosis did, inadvertently—I didn't know at the time," she explains, "is that it started me on a path that opened up numerous other doors. I doubt I would have become a social worker or gone into music therapy. I might have studied physical education only."

While looking at the big picture is something you ultimately have to do yourself, there are plenty of people who can help you along the way. Parents, teachers, friends, counseling professionals, and national and local scoliosis organizations are all sources of help.

Finding Support From Your Parents

Your parents are concerned about you. If you work together, parents can turn out to be your biggest source of support. Michelle Ann Mauney credits her father, a personal trainer, with helping her maintain the superb physical conditioning that made it possible for her to win her crown.

The trick, for both parents and kids, lies in maintaining a balance. Believe me, many parents worry about being too bossy, but somebody's got to be in charge. It is appropriate for parents to have a say in your life and in your scoliosis treatment. They are concerned with your welfare, although at times you may not believe it.

Does this mean you have no say at all in what happens to you? Absolutely not. Your cooperation is essential. It's your life, and your spine. No one can really impose a treatment plan on you and expect it to work unless you make it happen.

The more you understand, the more likely it is that you will follow through with a treatment plan. From the very first doctor's visit, you should be kept informed. If, after the visit, you don't understand why the doctor prescribed a particular course of treatment—a brace, for example— you should ask your parents to explain what the doctor told them. Maybe the whole family can sit down and watch a video about scoliosis and other spinal disorders. Ask any questions that trouble you, and if your parents don't know the answers, they can find out from the doctor or a scoliosis support group.

In addition to knowing the facts, you have a right to share your feelings. Don't keep them bottled up. Since scoliosis is often genetically transmitted, there's a good chance that your mother (or possibly your father) had a similar experience during adolescence. She will probably understand your emotions and be eager to help. Often just sharing your fear, anger, or bewilderment is the first step to making it go away.

Sharing your feelings isn't the same as making your parents give in to you. This is where the balancing act comes in. Carla Podzius puts it this way: "It's often a polarity: There are parents who force a child to take the treatment without explaining to the child what's going on. Then you have the opposite, where actually the child rules the parents.

"I've had experience with parents of a twelve-year-old daughter who were having difficulty because the daughter didn't want to talk about her scoliosis, didn't want to mention anything. When I called, I couldn't identify myself on the phone because she might hear the message. If I wrote to them, I couldn't put the stamp of the Scoliosis Association on the letter. None of her classmates knew. She wouldn't even talk to her brother about it. [There was a] big shroud of secrecy.

"So those are two polarities, two opposite sides. There has to be something in the middle that works to the healthy benefit of all concerned."

It is important for you to trust your parents and for them to listen to you and take your feelings into account. When you work together, you may find that your parents can give you much of the support you need.

Coping with Friends and Classmates

Very often kids pick on someone who looks different because they are afraid. It's part "I'm glad I don't look like that," and part "Maybe someday I could look like that."

Teasing is a problem for all kids, not just those with scoliosis. If a young person stands out in any way, he or she may become a target. If you're very smart or very tall, others may tease you out of envy. If you're short or can't understand math, they may tease you because they feel superior. No one likes to be teased, but kids who are really afraid of it and can't hide their fear are more likely to be the butt of jokes.

Scoliosis does not automatically open up a person for teasing. Many curves, especially lateral curves, are not easy for classmates to spot. If a teen has a pronounced rib hump or a kyphosis, it may be visible. More frequently, teens are teased if they wear braces. Almost all braces are visible through clothing, especially the Milwaukee brace , which includes a neck piece and a chin rest. The job of a brace is to hold the back rigid so that the curve won't progress. Therefore, the wearer will move somewhat stiffly and awkwardly.

I was teased terribly as a teenager, but never because I had scoliosis. I was intellectually ahead of my peers and socially behind them, so I was called a "brain" and an "egghead." But the main reason I was teased was that I showed how much I hated it. I cried a lot, and of course, the more they teased, the more I cried. The only time the teasing stopped was when I came back to school after scoliosis surgery, wearing a body cast. Maybe the other kids didn't want to pick on someone who was "down," but I suspect that my parents, teachers, and friends also made it clear that teasing wouldn't be tolerated. And this is a very important point.

As a teenager, you spend at least a third of your waking hours in school, so your school experience is bound to affect how you see yourself. For about six hours every day, five days of every week, teachers are the adults with whom you interact.

A teacher can be a tremendous help to a student who is struggling with problems. By the time you're in junior high or high school, you see a number of different teachers in the course of a day, so even if you and your homeroom teacher have nothing in common, you may relate well to your gym teacher or your English teacher. But no one can help unless he or she knows there is a problem.

If you feel self-conscious, or if you really are being picked on, see if you can arrange to speak to a favorite teacher or school counselor for ten minutes. At the very least, he or she can serve as a sounding board. At best, teachers can suggest strategies for dealing with a troublesome classmate.

Education may help to minimize the teasing. Try speaking with the school nurse or your physical education teacher. Perhaps they would agree to devote some class time to talking about scoliosis and related spinal problems. Many good videos are available that clearly explain the difficulties. (See the For Further Reading section at the end of the book.) Once your classmates are more knowledgeable about what you are dealing with, they may stop seeing you as someone to be teased and see you as they did before—as another friend and classmate

Role playing can help. You and your parents can play-act possible scenarios, taking different parts—a kid with a brace, the class bully, a friend, a teacher. Role playing can show you your options in reacting to a situation. Trying to figure out what other people think of scoliosis may help you understand why people act a certain way or say hurtful things. This understanding may help you to stop feeling like a victim and may make it easier to use your sense of humor to disarm others with laughter. Role playing now can help you to be in control when a difficult situation arises in the future.

Another good strategy is to talk with your teachers and friends and tell them about the situation in advance. If you are shy about telling your best friend that you're going to have to wear a back brace, sit down with your parents and plan how to say it. It's very important to be able to communicate.

By discussing your fears in advance ("I'm afraid classmates will tease me once I start wearing a brace"), teachers and parents may help you avoid difficult situations. They can help you size things up. Which kid or kids are you afraid of? Why do you think they will pick on you? What can you say to avoid a bad situation or in response to an unkind comment? Who are your friends and how can they help?

Try not to make your scoliosis a deep, dark secret. Keeping your scoliosis a secret can only make your tension and fears seem worse. Talking about it helps.

There's Help Out There

Scoliosis and other spinal disorders sometimes can seem overwhelming. You think your life has been going along pretty well and you've been happy. Then something suddenly comes along that turns your world upside down. You may have to wear a brace or have surgery and, for a while at least, you may not be able to participate in many of the activities you've always enjoyed. Life seems to be falling apart. Your parents and teachers try to help, but they really don't understand, or so you think. What do you do?

It's no disgrace to seek outside help. If you don't know of

a local support group, write the Scoliosis Association, Inc., for the address of the chapter nearest you. Both parents and teenagers can find support at a meeting of the association. Cindy Soldatich is the youth group director of the association's Long Island chapter. Soldatich, now in her twenties, was diagnosed with scoliosis at sixteen. She runs group sessions for girls ages six to seventeen, discussing "friends, movies, family vacations, camp, and school," among other topics. A boy may attend an occasional meeting, but usually it's just girls. "Our meetings offer support and a place to talk about feelings," Cindy says. "The girls feel comfortable talking to each other and discussing what other members are going through."

If this kind of informal peer-group support doesn't do the trick, there's nothing wrong with seeking one-on-one help. A school guidance counselor or psychologist can help. Or your parents may seek an outside counselor for individual or family counseling. Carla Podzius counsels both children with scoliosis and their parents, individually or together. The local Scoliosis Association may be able to recommend someone. Or your orthopedist or scoliosis specialist can point you to a mental health professional who works to help scoliosis patients feel good about themselves.

It's no disgrace to ask for professional help. In fact, it's a sign of maturity. Often, you need just a session or two with someone who can be objective and who is not personally involved in your problems, to help you gain perspective and deal with your feelings about scoliosis and its treatment. If the counselor is familiar with scoliosis, that's a plus. The main thing is that it's got to be someone you trust, to whom you can open up and who will listen.

A Look in the Mirror

So far we've been looking at self-image, how we see our-selves from the inside, our mental picture of ourselves. What about the physical picture—the person each of us sees when we look in a mirror? We can't really separate the two, of course: how we look influences how we feel about ourselves, and vice versa.

Even if no one else can see that you have scoliosis, sco-liosis can make you feel awkward and unattractive. One shoulder may be higher than the other, your waistline diagonal instead of straight across, and the hems of skirts crooked. Often no one notices it but you. There are many small adjustments you may want to try to make your appearance one with which you are happy.

Michelle Ann Mauney speaks to teens around the coun-try about improving their motivation and self-image. One of the services she offers is fashion consulting. "I work with everybody," she says, "but I do see a lot of girls who have scoliosis or other back deformities. If they have a problem with the hips, or if their shoulders are uneven, you have to improvise. There are lots of little tricks. As far as the design, you want to take the emphasis away from the curvature and focus the eye elsewhere. You work with shoulder pads; you may want to put two on one side and one on the other. I advise girls to have their clothes altered to fit them. Many times, clothes off the rack will not fit a person with scoliosis."

A skilled tailor or dressmaker can really help a person with scoliosis. He knows how to make one pants leg shorter than the other to make the pants appear even. She can adjust a skirt hem to accommodate a curvature, even if it means making the skirt two or three inches shorter on one side than the other. This is almost impossible to do by yourself. If you are very skilled with a needle, have a friend help you mark the garment while you try it on and then hem it yourself. Many people with scoliosis, however, prefer to buy fewer clothes but allow room in the clothing budget for professional tailoring.

Avoid buying clothes with horizontal or vertical stripes. Girls should also avoid straight skirts with a center seam or slit. No matter how you try to alter it, the seam will form a diagonal, pointing at one of your knees instead of the floor. Plaids can pose a challenge, but here a skilled dressmaker can usually help, especially with a fairly long, full skirt. A sharply defined waistline may also call attention to your scoliosis.

A little creativity can help you get around these obstacles. Try buying clothes with diagonal stripes. It sounds wild, but I had a diagonally striped dress once, and it never failed to attract compliments. The stripes do an excellent job of disguising the curvature. Experiment with colored and printed fabrics that call attention to your assets.

Look for dresses without conventional waistlines. "A-line" models with lots of soft fabric look and feel very good. A dropped waistline is all right, as long as it doesn't call attention to uneven hips. An Empire waist, just below the bustline, has an effect similar to that of the A-line. Overblouses are great with pants and skirts. They conceal an uneven waistline and are attractive and comfortable. If you like wearing belts, try making a slit in each side seam of your A-line dress or overblouse. You can pull the belt through in front but leave the back loose. This gives a tailored look without calling attention to an uneven waist.

Hems don't have to be a problem, as long as you avoid straight, tight skirts. Soft, full skirts are very attractive. The long, flowered skirts that are so popular today are ideal. "Handkerchief hems," which have a lot of little points around the hemline, are very flattering. If the hem is meant to be irregular, or if it's around your ankles, people are less likely to notice your scoliosis.

At one time, I had to wear a lift in one shoe to compensate for the difference in leg length caused by the scoliosis. Some doctors and physical therapists continue to recommend lifts, which do seem to help some people. The lift is usually a simple pad placed inside the heel of the shoe. It can be worn with any low- or medium-heeled shoe, so you don't have to wear "orthopedic" shoes just because you have scoliosis. I wouldn't recommend stiletto heels or three-inch platforms for anyone, but teens with scoliosis don't have to wear special shoes. Any comfortable shoe that provides good support is fine.

As I said earlier, how you look influences how you feel, and vice versa. If you work on feeling good about yourself—"accentuate the positive," as the old song says—you'll look better, too. So keep your chin up, literally and figuratively. Remember, scoliosis is not only part of the growth process, it's also a growth experience.

Bracing for the Best

When Christine was nine years old, her pediatrician noticed that her back was irregular. Her shoulders and hips were even, but when Christine bent over, the doctor noticed a "high back," or rib hump, on one side. An X ray confirmed a thoracic (upper) curve of about 25 degrees and a 32-degree lumbar (lower) curve.

The curve was significant, but not enormous. Had Christine been in her late teens, with little growing left to do, the doctor might have said, "Let's wait and see." But Christine was only nine, and in six or seven years, a 32-degree curve could easily become a 60-degree curve. The doctor told Christine and her parents that she should start wearing a brace right away.

Christine found the brace difficult to contend with at first. "In the beginning, everyone at school knew about my brace and they made a big deal about it. They called me names," Christine said. Despite the teasing, she continued to wear her brace because the doctor told her it was the only way to avoid surgery. It didn't stop her from taking part in sports. The doctor let her take it off for swimming, as long as she agreed to put it on as soon as she got out of the water.

"She's a real trooper, but she has her down moments," said Christine's mother. For six years Christine has worn the brace. It hasn't stopped her from growing into a normal, happy teenager or from being very active in drama club, her favorite extracurricular activity.

I spoke with Christine when she was sixteen. She would soon be done with the brace. "They are going to start weaning me off the brace in two months," she told me. "I've stopped growing, but the growth plate hasn't fully closed yet." Although the weaning process would take time, she sounded happy to see the light at the end of the tunnel.

"What would you tell a ten-year-old who was facing six years of brace-wearing?" I asked her.

"Just stick with it," Christine said, "When you get older, the brace will come off. It's worth it in the long run."

What Is a Brace?

In the Middle Ages, back braces, heavy metal corsets for people with scoliosis, were made by armorers, the same craftsmen who equipped knights for battle. The idea was that the brace would hold the spine rigid and prevent the scoliosis from progressing. Only the wealthy could afford them, and they must have been very uncomfortable.

Although these medieval braces did not succeed, the idea of creating an external structure to support the spine and prevent curve progression has persisted since the earliest days of medicine. More progress has been made in brace development during the past fifty years than in all the preceding centuries.

A brace, or orthosis (straightener), is an appliance made of plastic and/or metal that is designed to support a young person's spine and prevent the curve from progressing. Braces are recommended for children and teens whose bones are in the process of growing. Once full skeletal maturity has been achieved, doctors seldom recommend braces to arrest scoliosis, although they may prescribe a brace to support the healing spine after surgery.

Braces don't just support the back. They actually force the spine into a straighter position. Through the use of pads held in place by metal supports, pressure is applied on the curve to make it straighten out. Most currently available braces have some kind of pads, which are held in place by the brace's metal rods and plastic plates. However, the first "modern" brace, the Milwaukee brace, also has a neck ring, which exerts a pull on the spine from the top. This kind of brace is often described as "active" or "dynamic," because of its push-me, pull-you effects on the spine. It became even more active when the wearer used the neck ring and other parts of the brace to perform a series of exercises. The combination of brace and exercises was designed to develop the muscles of the upper body to help hold the curve straight after the brace was removed.

The so-called low-profile braces currently in favor do contain pads that exert pressure on the spine, but while lower, they are also more solid than the Milwaukee brace, which is made up of plastic sections connected by metal rods with considerable space between. As a result, the newer braces are often called "passive" or "static," because their main function is to hold the spine in a straighter position, not to make it "active."

In 1946, when the Milwaukee brace was developed, it was hailed as a breakthrough in scoliosis treatment because it combined support with active correction. Today, many physicians still believe that a dynamic brace is far better than a passive one. Others, including some of the leaders in scoliosis treatment, say the Milwaukee brace is not significantly more effective than passive braces. Whether this is because the brace is not the miracle it was once thought to be, or because it is difficult to get a teenager to wear it, is still a matter of debate.

Bracing Works

Wearing a brace can be a pain in the neck—sometimes literally. The good news is that bracing works—not for every person every time, but for many people. For kids who are diagnosed and treated at a young age, like Christine, a brace can often stem the progression of scoliosis and prevent the need for surgery.

"As sure as the sun will come up in the morning, braces are effective," said Dr. Alf Nachemson, as quoted in the National Scoliosis Foundation Newsletter. Dr. Nachemson lives in Gothenburg, Sweden, and was the principal investigator in a study sponsored by the Scoliosis Research Society. Nachemson and his colleagues in medical centers throughout the world followed the progress of almost 300 girls with adolescent idiopathic scoliosis. One hundred thirty-one patients in five centers were not given braces, while 115 patients in three other centers were. After five years, curves in 70 percent of the nonbraced patients had progressed 6 degrees or more, in contrast to only 20 percent of the braced ones.

Bracing works only if curves are detected fairly early and if the patient hasn't reached skeletal maturity. Nachemson's study is one reason that the National Scoliosis Foundation and other advocates recommend school screening.

Although wearing a brace can prevent a curve from getting worse, most orthopedists agree that it doesn't make the curve go away. However, if a person's scoliosis is like Christine's, with one curve in the high twenties and another in the low or middle thirties, that can be enough. Initially, Christine's scoliosis was so mild that the school nurse did not find it during a routine screening just two months earlier. The doctor didn't even see it until she bent over. People with such curves can live long and happy lives with scoliosis, as long as it doesn't get worse.

Even if there's a chance that in the future the curve will get worse and surgery will be recommended, doctors often try a brace first. If the curve is between 25 and 40 degrees and doesn't get worse, surgery can probably be avoided. If it does get worse, there's still time to decide whether to have surgery. While doctors sometimes operate on very young children with severe scoliosis, they generally prefer to wait until growth slows down or stops. In the meantime, it's not a bad idea to try to stop the curve from getting worse by using a brace.

Basic Bracing from Milwaukee

The idea of bracing a back to keep it from curving is not new. It's logical to want to prop something up if it's leaning over—like tying a young plant to a wooden stake to make

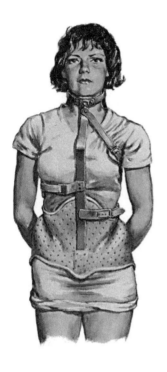 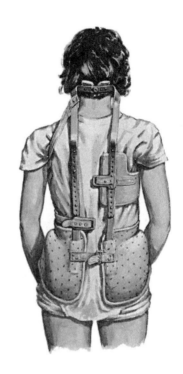

The Milwaukee brace, seen from the side (left) and back (right). Unlike many newer types of braces, the Milwaukee brace is an active brace—it exerts a pull on the spine while also holding it in a straight position.

it grow upright. Hippocrates not only gave scoliosis its name, he also tried to correct it with an early form of bracing. Over the centuries, doctors have used all kinds of devices to try to straighten up a crooked spine.

In *Deenie*, noted author Judy Blume wrote about a girl who is diagnosed with scoliosis and has to wear a back brace. Initially she is very upset, but she discovers that she is the same person with the brace as she is without.

The brace Deenie wore was the Milwaukee brace,

developed in 1945 by Drs. Walter Blount and Albert Schmidt of the Medical College of Wisconsin and Milwaukee's Children's Hospital. Dr. Schmidt was an engineer as well as a doctor. He and Dr. Blount first developed the brace to take the place of a cast following scoliosis surgery. At that time, most doctors assumed that braces could not be used to correct or halt scoliosis. Surgery seemed to be the only option. In the past, braces had unintentionally weakened muscles.

The Milwaukee brace turned out to be even better than Drs. Schmidt and Blount had hoped. They discovered that it worked well both for postoperative patients and as an alternative treatment to surgery.

The Milwaukee brace has been streamlined since its invention, but the principle hasn't changed. It's a strange-looking contraption. The first thing most kids notice about the brace is that it shows above their clothing. A neck ring or throat mold is used to center the head above the pelvis, and this shows above shirts. Centering the head immediately makes the spine straighter. The rest of the brace is made up of a plastic pelvic piece to which one frontal and two rear metal uprights are connected. The rear uprights go all the way up the back and connect with the neck ring. Attached to the sides of the rear uprights are pads that push on the curve and try to prevent it from worsening.

The Milwaukee brace is considered an "active" brace. People wearing the brace can—and should—exercise while wearing it. This keeps their muscles strong, helping the correction to hold after the brace is removed.

According to Dr. Blount, "To be successful, passive cor-

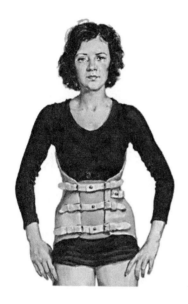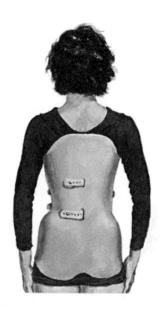

The low-profile brace shown here is used for curves that start in the chest area and end below the waist (thoracolumbar curves) or for curves in the lower back area (lumbar curves).

rection by the brace needs to be combined with active movements of the patient and ideally with a few simple specific exercises."

I asked Dr. Lubicky, of Chicago Shriner's Hospital, how he convinces children and teenagers to wear the Milwaukee brace.

"I approach bracing in a reasonable manner," he said. "For example, I tell them they can take regular gym without the brace. That allows them to do everything. Also, in the summertime I tell them, 'If you want to go swimming, fine. Just take the brace off and go swimming. That doesn't mean you can lie around the pool without the brace, but go swimming as much as you want.' That's how I try to get them to look at it in a positive way. I tell them, 'The brace is your friend. Your friend is trying to prevent you from having an operation. And you have to do the best you can.'"

Deenie wore a Milwaukee brace because there weren't many alternatives in 1973. Today many other braces are available.

Keeping a Low Profile

When Kristin Zachmann was six years old, she was diagnosed with juvenile scoliosis. While doctors may disagree about how effective braces are for adolescent scoliosis, they agree that braces frequently help juvenile scoliosis patients, children twelve and under. Kristin was given a Boston brace.

The Boston brace is one of a number of braces called TLSOs, short for thoracic (upper back) lumbar (middle back) sacral (lower back) orthoses (braces). Since both "thoracic lumbar sacral orthosis" and "TLSO" are a mouthful, most people call these "low-profile" braces or use the name of the city where the brace was developed.

The Boston brace was designed by Dr. John Hall and Bill Miller of Boston Children's Hospital in the 1970s. Other low-profile braces include the Wilmington and Miami braces and the European Ponte, Riviera, and Lyon versions.

Low-profile braces, which go from under the arms to the hips, are less noticeable than the Milwaukee brace. Many teens with low-profile braces wear oversized T-shirts, which often camouflage the brace.

Low-profile braces can be custom-made by an orthotist

(brace-maker). The majority of low-profile braces use ready-made plastic molds that the orthotist customizes for each person. On the inside of the brace are the pads that push on the curve. The braces open in back or in front.

Sara-Marie Stefanski's curvature was discovered when she was eleven. Because the X rays showed only an 18-degree curve, the doctor decided to wait and see. "If the curve progresses beyond 30 degrees, we'll have to use a brace," he said.

The curve did progress, and Sara-Marie now wears a Boston brace. When I interviewed her, she was fifteen and wearing the brace twenty-three hours a day. Her curve had not progressed beyond 31 degrees. When she reaches sixteen, her physician plans to start weaning her from the brace by gradually reducing the number of hours she will wear it.

To Sara-Marie, wearing the brace is no big deal. A few of her friends know she wears it, and they don't make a fuss. She is allowed to take it off for gymnastics, which she enjoys. She sees her doctor every four months for follow-up.

Kristin Zachmann, now a teenager, wears her brace only twelve hours a day. Her curvature has progressed, but only from 35 to 38 degrees. Although she doesn't wear it to school, her friends know about it, and their only reaction is curiosity. "When they ask me how it is, whether it feels comfortable, I say, 'It's okay, you know, but it's something you have to live with,'" Kristin told me.

Traditionally, doctors have asked that braces be worn twenty-three hours a day. It takes a few days to get used to a brace. For many wearers, the brace becomes like a second skin after a while.

Recently, doctors like Kristin's have been prescribing

braces for less than twenty-three hours a day—twelve in Kristin's case, but more commonly sixteen. Wearers can go to school without it, providing they put it on as soon as they come home. They must also sleep in it.

"I know all the tricks," Dr. Lubicky said to me. "Teens go out of the house through the garage, leave the brace in the garage, and go to school. Then they come home through the garage, put the brace back on, and hope that their mother thinks they wore the brace all day."

Bending the Rules

The Charleston bending brace was developed in 1979. This particular brace is designed to be worn only at night while the patient is asleep. It is molded to conform to the wearer's body while she is bending toward the convex (rounded) side of her curve, "overcorrecting" the scoliosis. The theory is that overcorrecting for eight hours a day might have the same effect as correcting for twenty-three.

To understand how the brace works, think of a wall poster rolled into a mailing tube for shipping or a diploma rolled up and tied with a ribbon. Before framing the poster or diploma, you roll it up in the opposite direction. When you've done this a few times, the paper straightens out.

The Charleston bending brace forces wearers to bend over to one side, in the opposite direction from the way their spines curve. It would be extremely difficult to walk, sit, or stand in this position for any length of time, but it is not difficult to sleep this way. Some teens who refuse to wear a brace during the day raise fewer objections to wearing one at night.

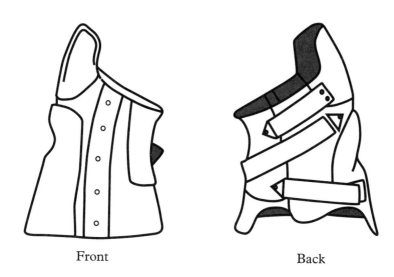

Front   Back

The Charleston bending brace, designed to be worn while sleeping.

Some physicians are skeptical about this brace. They do not think wearing any brace for only eight hours can be effective. However, the National Scoliosis Foundation has reported, "A preliminary study and subsequent longer-term follow-up of those using the nighttime bending brace are encouraging, particularly for a single curve." To date, there has not been enough reliable long-term research to prove whether the Charleston brace is as effective as other braces.

Is That All There Is?

The Milwaukee brace, various low-profile models, and the newer Charleston bending brace are the braces used most often by the majority of orthopedists who specialize in scoliosis treatment.

The Copes Scoliosis Total Recovery System (TRS) is a controversial treatment for scoliosis. Founded by orthotist Arthur L. Copes, the system claims not just to stop the curve from progressing as other braces do but to correct scoliosis. The cornerstone of this system is the Copes Dynamic Brace, an air-injected brace that is made to fit close to the skin and, therefore, be unnoticeable to others. With the Copes Dynamic Brace, the neck ring of the Milwaukee brace has been eliminated. The Copes Dynamic Brace is also less rigid than the Boston and other low-profile braces. Through the application of air pressure to the curved area, the brace is said to "gently encourage curvature correction."

The brace is only part of the Copes TRS, which includes electronic muscle stimulation, exercise, chiropractic care, nutritional therapy, and hydrotherapy. Some of these treatments, including the electronic muscle stimulation, have no proven effect on scoliosis. A healthy diet is certainly important, but it cannot "fix" a curved spine.

The Copes system has aroused strong feelings on both sides. Daniel Brotschul is a satisfied Copes customer. "I am a twenty-three-year-old male who has suffered from progressive idiopathic scoliosis since early childhood," he writes. "By the time I reached mid-adolescence, my double curve was so severe [that] I was unable to sit, stand, or sleep without great effort. At the age of sixteen, I wore the Copes brace for three years, in conjunction with other therapies, to address the various muscular, skeletal, and neurological problems that contribute to scoliosis. I have been completely corrected and without pain for about five years, and my spine has been stabilized without surgery." Daniel and his family chose the brace themselves.

Not all Copes users echo Daniel's enthusiasm. Some teens are disappointed to find that the brace is not as inconspicuous as its makers claim, and that it does in fact show through their clothing. One young man complained of the difficulties of fitting all the elements of the TRS—exercises, bath therapy, chiropractic visits, etc.—into a busy school schedule. Yet Copes proponents claim the brace is effective only if used in conjunction with the TRS.

To date, it appears that controlled clinical trials, the accepted scientific method of testing new treatments and appliances, have not been used to evaluate the Copes TRS, or if such trials have been done, it is extremely difficult to find the results. It would be interesting to see how well the Copes brace functioned in conjunction with a more conventional bracing program or to evaluate the other elements of the TRS using another kind of brace. It appears unlikely, however, that such a clinical trial protocol will be developed in the near future.

You may want to ask your doctor about the Copes TRS. However, your orthopedist cannot prescribe the brace, which must be used in conjunction with the complete program, or the system. Instead, you must consult a participating chiropractor, and only select chiropractors use the system.

It is important to note that the Scoliosis Research Society, the orthopedic group that specializes in spinal deformities, does not endorse the Copes TRS. Some insurance carriers will not cover this system, which, while much less costly than surgery, is expensive.

Other "nonsurgical" treatments for scoliosis surface from time to time, often through the Internet. It's a good idea not to enroll in any program until you check with your doctor. Also, find out what the program or appliance will cost and whether your family's insurance will cover it.

Living With a Brace

Talking with Christine, Kristin, and Sara-Marie, I became convinced that wearing a brace isn't the worst thing in the world. All three girls have adjusted to their braces and don't let it rule their lives. All three have supportive mothers and families.

That doesn't mean wearing a brace isn't a hassle sometimes. Even after the initial period of adjustment, there are times when all brace wearers would like to be free. It's natural to feel awkward from time to time and to envy other kids who seem to be able to do everything more easily. Brace wearers have to learn new ways of bending over. Milwaukee brace wearers can't bend their necks well, so they often have to study at standing desks or counters, or put their books on a stand in front of them.

If you have problems or questions about wearing a brace, don't hesitate to draw on all the resources I mentioned in the previous chapter: your parents, teachers, counselors, friends, and scoliosis support groups. You may also want to do further research to determine the best course of action. Reach out for help; it's there for you.

Getting Fitted

When I was a teenager, I became very friendly with Jack and Miss Kay in the brace shop of the hospital where my orthopedist practiced. I didn't know that Jack, and possibly Miss Kay as well, was an "orthotist."

An orthotist is trained to make appliances that straighten deformities. It is important that your brace be fitted by a skilled orthotist. Most spine centers contain an orthotics department with highly trained practitioners, although some do use orthotists who have their own facilities outside the hospital.

The orthopedist writes a prescription for a brace, either to be made of prefabricated parts and adjusted to fit the patient's curve, or custom-made. Either option is fine, but a customized prefabricated brace usually works well, especially in the case of low-profile braces.

If the doctor prescribes a brace for you, you'll be sent to an orthotist, who will take various measurements in the area to be covered by the brace. You may want to take your X rays to the orthotist in addition to the prescription. The more information the orthotist has, the better the brace will be.

If it's a prefabricated brace, the orthotist will pick a mold from stock and adapt it to your size and shape by cutting and trimming it and using a heat gun to change the shape of the plastic, if necessary. Pads are then attached to the inside of the brace to exert pressure on the curve.

For a custom-made brace, the orthotist will make a plaster cast of your torso, carefully remove it from you, fill it with liquid plaster to make an exact replica of your trunk area, and then remove the cast. The brace is then molded on this plaster model. When you come back for a fitting, the brace is adapted to fit you, much the same way as with prefabricated braces. I've had a low-profile brace custom-made, and I remember the time and care that the orthotist devoted to me, making sure the brace conformed to the doctor's prescription and was as comfortable as it could possibly be.

Both low-profile and Milwaukee braces are made this way—either from prefabricated parts or from scratch.

Brace Couture—High and Low

What you wear under a brace can make a difference. Braces, especially the low-profile ones, are made of solid, rigid plastic. They are static braces. The Milwaukee brace contains both metal and plastic and is a dynamic brace.

Neither kind of brace should be worn next to the skin. The rigid plastic will rub the skin, and because plastic doesn't 'breathe,' it will be extremely hot. You should wear a form-fitting undergarment—a tube top or sleeveless undershirt—under the brace. This should be made of cotton, preferably 100 percent, but at least 65 percent. Cotton absorbs perspiration, unlike synthetic fibers, which can leave perspiration trapped between the undershirt and the body. It's important that your undershirt fits you exactly. If it's too loose, it will wrinkle and cause chafing. If it's too short, the bottom of the brace will rub against your hipbones, and that hurts.

Since fit is so important, you may want to order undershirts specially designed to fit under braces. See the

Where to Go for Help section at the end of this book for ordering information. Underclothes made for wearing with braces are not cheap, but many medical insurance policies cover the cost.

Store-bought undershirts may work fine. They may stretch after a number of washings, but they can be easily replaced. If you do order the custom-made kind, be sure to order a fairly large supply. You'll want to wash them after every wearing, especially in summer. And they may stretch or wear out after a while, so you'll need to keep some in reserve.

Some people experience skin irritation under the brace, at least at first. Usually, this goes away as your skin becomes accustomed to the brace. It's important not to use lotions, powders, or creams under a brace, as they soften and moisten the skin, making it more likely to develop sores if the brace rubs against it. You may want to use rubbing alcohol to soothe roughened areas. If the problem persists, the brace may not fit properly. Check with your doctor.

What you wear over a brace is important in terms of your state of mind. Don't let your loose-fitting clothing make you see yourself as fat or unattractive. Use the fact that you have to buy new clothes as an opportunity to be creative. Try new color schemes and fabrics. You may find that your brace pokes holes in your clothing from time to time, so don't get anything too expensive. Nice-looking, inexpensive overblouses or turtlenecks don't have to be costly, and if they wear out, you can get more. Treat yourself to a pretty new scarf or two and, for special occasions, a new party dress or pants outfit.

Shaping Up with a Brace

In addition to the orthopedist who prescribes the brace and the orthotist who constructs it, physical therapists are often an important part of the team that works with scoliosis patients.

Braces do keep scoliosis curves straight, but they may have some undesirable side effects, like allowing certain muscles to soften up or flattening out the natural lordosis (the bottom part of the front-to-back curve). This is particularly true of the low-profile braces. To strengthen muscles the brace could otherwise weaken, the physical therapist will prescribe exercises and show you how to do them.

Marisela Gonzalez is a physical therapist who was formerly with the Scoliosis Program at St. Vincent's Medical Center in New York City.

"We involved kids who wear braces in an exercise program," Gonzalez said. "There is nothing in the literature that says physical therapy or exercise will cure scoliosis," she continued, "but it certainly helps [delay the] progression of the curvature."

Gonzalez believes kids who wear braces and do exercises faithfully can avoid surgery. "That's the ultimate goal," she explained. "When kids came to the program to find out whether they needed surgery, the doctor often recommended a brace and exercises first, in hopes that they would not have to have surgery." The program is fairly new, but so far the kids who had come for therapy and worn a brace have not had surgery.

Gonzalez asked teens to come in three times a week to

do the exercises with her. She tailored the exercises to fit the teens—not only what they needed, but how much they could be expected to do. Strengthening stomach muscles, preserving the normal lordosis, and increasing flexibility are among the goals of physical therapy for the scoliosis patient who wears a brace.

If you think wearing a brace will get you out of gym class, think again. Physical therapists and orthopedists agree that it's important for teens to stay active when they wear braces. If you wear a brace for only twelve or sixteen hours a day, you will already have it off for gym. The doctor may ask you not to engage in really rough contact sports. As for gymnastics and skiing, sports that involve twisting, it really depends on your doctor and your level of expertise. The doctor won't want you to twist too much because you might injure your back. However, if you're an expert skier, he or she may let you ski—with the brace on for protection.

Checkups and Changes

After I had worn a brace for six months, it began to rub against my left hip constantly. Since I was due for a checkup, I made an appointment to see the orthopedist immediately.

"Doctor, why is the brace rubbing?" I asked. "It never did this before."

His answer was reassuring. The brace was doing its job. My scoliosis had shifted, only slightly, but enough to make my hip, once almost flat, now protrude slightly. My waistline was becoming less slanted, the other hip less protruding.

You shouldn't panic if your brace becomes uncomfortable. It may prove that your brace is also doing its job. You do need regular checkups to monitor your scoliosis. Since braces are usually prescribed only for kids who are growing, most young people need a new brace every year or two. The average life of a brace is fifteen months. Most kids will have to wear a brace for a minimum of two or three years and as long as seven or eight.

During the first year, you'll visit the orthopedist fairly frequently. This is usually just to see how you are adjusting and if you have any problems or questions. After that, you'll see the orthopedist to check on your progress and the orthotist to adjust the brace or get a new one.

Freedom—A Gradual Process

As teens approach skeletal maturity, their bone growth starts to slow down. Although I keep talking about the ages of sixteen for girls and eighteen for boys, those are just averages. Doctors look at measurements such as the Risser scale and the filling in of the growth plates to gauge skeletal maturity for each person.

For example, if a girl is fifteen, got her first period at fourteen, and measures three on the Risser scale, the doctor may assume her growth rate is slowing down. The doctor will then ask the girl to come in to the office after she's been out of the brace eight hours. If the curve measures the same as it did the last time he X-rayed her, when she was wearing the brace full-time (twenty-three hours a day), the doctor may let her spend eight hours or nine hours of every day out of the brace. For the next checkup, he may let her take the brace off for twelve hours. Then

108

she may have to wear the brace only when sleeping. Doing away with the brace entirely isn't recommended until full skeletal maturity is reached.

This is the "weaning" process Christine and Sara-Marie are looking forward to. Christine's doctor is confident that she won't need any more treatment than perhaps an occasional checkup. Sara-Marie's doctor has been a little more cautious. He said if the brace doesn't work, she might need surgery. However, with the curvature holding at 31 degrees, things are looking good. If the curvature doesn't progress after the brace comes off, Sara-Marie can enjoy a happy, active life, including her beloved gymnastics.

Does scoliosis ever progress after bone maturity has been achieved? Orthopedists used to say never or very rarely. Now they have found that some curves do progress in adulthood. The worse the curve, the more likely it is to progress. Curves of over 50 degrees have a good chance of progression, while curves of over 30 degrees have some chance. So Sara-Marie's curve might get worse after she matures, but the chances are good that it won't.

What happens to those kids whose curves are too bad to brace, or for whom bracing doesn't work? For a small percentage of scoliosis patients, surgery may be the best solution. Scoliosis surgery isn't as bad as it sounds, once you learn more about it.

The Big Decision

When Sara Rubin was ten years old and found out she had scoliosis, her curvature had already advanced to 35 degrees. For her age, that was a fairly large curve, so an orthopedist immediately pre-scribed a Wilmington low-profile brace, to be worn twenty-two hours a day.

Sara wore the brace for two years, but the curve kept getting bigger. By the time she was twelve, it was 50 degrees. The doctor recommended spinal fusion surgery—changing a portion of the spine from a series of segments (vertebrae) into a solid bone—to correct the problem. Scoliosis surgery is generally some form of spinal fusion.

Sara was fifteen when I interviewed her. The surgery had been successful; the curve was "25 degrees and holding." The two scars on her back are exposed when she wears a bathing suit, but she doesn't mind too much. Asked what she would tell teens faced with the prospect of surgery, she says, "I'd tell them it does hurt, but the pain goes away. It's better than a brace. If I had a brace, I would still be wearing it."

After two years of "watchful waiting," Alicia Peterman was given a Boston brace to stabilize her S-curve, which measured 25 degrees on top and 21 degrees at the bottom. In ninth grade, she wore the brace under baggy clothes. In tenth grade, she admits, she didn't wear it.

"The brace became a social problem for her," Alicia's mother says. "It ended up under her bed more than on her body." At sixteen, Alicia underwent a spinal fusion.

Five months after the surgery, Alicia's mother said, "She is feeling and looking very good. She is more outgoing and talkative now, and has a better mental attitude." After her one-year checkup, Alicia's curves had been reduced to a mere 16 and 20 degrees. Her surgeon said the fusion was healing nicely and that there were no restrictions on her physical activity. Alicia has to see her doctor every six months, but otherwise, she's free to be a teenager and forget about the operation.

Samantha Fish wore a brace for two years, but she had surgery twice. In 1992, when she was twelve and a half, her chest wall began to collapse, so surgery could not be delayed. Three years later, Samantha had grown five inches, and a second operation was needed. When I spoke to her in June 1997, Samantha said, "Everything is perfect. Everyone comments on how good my posture is. I can do everything I want in school. I was on kick line. I can even do some gymnastics if I want to."

Michael Buff never wore a brace. His scoliosis was treated with "watchful waiting" until he was fifteen. Then doctors told him that "since I was a man, a brace would most likely not work. I would have to have one until I was eighteen and then probably have surgery. So I just said, 'Oh, let's get it over with.'" When I interviewed Michael, who is now thirty-two, he spoke of scoliosis as a thing of the past. "I barely remember to go for my checkups," he admitted. His back doesn't bother him and he considers the operation a resounding success.

A Brief Description of Surgery

Historically, the surgeon performing a spinal fusion made an incision in the patient's back; this is called a posterior approach. In recent years, surgeons have also used an anterior approach.

Anterior means from the front, but the incision is usually made from the side of the body. The posterior approach is still used in most fusions of the upper or thoracic spine, but many physicians like the anterior approach for curves that start in the thoracic area and go to the lower or lumbar spine (thoracolumbar curves) or for lumbar curves. By doing the procedure from the front, the surgeon can do shorter fusions and obtain a better correction of the curve.

When surgeons use the anterior approach, they frequently remove a rib in order to gain access to the spine. The rib is then used for bone grafts for the spine, eliminating the need to take bone from elsewhere in the body. In some cases, surgeons use both the anterior and posterior approaches.

During surgery, physicians add "hardware," usually metal systems that hold the spine rigid and allow it to heal in place.

Why Choose Surgery?

For each of the four individuals mentioned above, surgery has provided some answers. My own experience with surgery was also a positive one. Still, no one denies that orthopedic surgery is a long, complicated process and should not be taken lightly.

Why do doctors recommend surgery for scoliosis? Why do patients and families choose a costly, painful, and time-consuming procedure? There are some forms of scoliosis for which surgery appears to be the best solution. A neuromuscular disease called neurofibromatosis can produce severe curvatures of the spine. Surgery is often the only answer for this type of curvature. When it comes to idiopathic scoliosis, however, it's legitimate to proceed with caution.

Surgery is the only method that has been scientifically proven to correct a spinal curvature, as opposed to bracing, which can arrest a curve and keep it from getting worse but cannot correct it. Doctors can't give you a perfectly straight spine, but they can make it much straighter. At "25 degrees and holding," Sara's scoliosis is definitely within acceptable limits. It's less than the 35 degrees she started with at age ten, and much less than the 50 degrees to which it had progressed.

For most doctors, 50 degrees is the magic number. If a curve progresses to 50 degrees before a child reaches skeletal maturity, there's a better-than-average chance that it will continue to deteriorate. If, in addition to the side-to-side curve getting worse, the vertebrae continue to rotate, heart and breathing problems could well develop later in life.

For many years, doctors mistakenly thought that scoliosis never progressed after full bone growth was achieved. Then a research study was done that followed scoliosis patients for a forty-year period. In two-thirds of the

patients, there was some scoliosis progression after skeletal maturity. Not surprisingly, the largest curves—those of
more than 50 degrees—had the greatest risk of progression. Curves of less than 30 degrees had almost no risk.

In my case, the doctors were more concerned with my
lumbar curve, which was significant, than the thoracic
one, which was comparatively minor. They warned that I
might have complications in pregnancy if the lumbar
curve were not corrected. Today, doctors find that relatively few scoliosis patients have difficulties in childbirth
because of lumbar curves, but women with lumbar curves
can experience an increase in lower back pain during
pregnancy.

Sometimes a doctor will recommend surgery for a 40-
degree curve. If a curve seems to have grown rapidly and
already exceeds 40 degrees but is not yet 50 degrees,
surgery may be a good idea. It depends on the location of
the curve, the age of the patient, the degree of rotation,
and other factors. Most surgeons seldom recommend
surgery for less than 40 degrees and usually recommend it
above 50—at least for teens—but there is considerable
variation from doctor to doctor and from case to case.

If a patient is experiencing severe back pain as a direct
result of scoliosis, doctors may ask her and her family to
consider surgery. However, teenagers almost never have
pain with a curvature. The absence of pain is the main
reason so many cases of adolescent scoliosis go undetected. Pain is much more of a consideration with adults,
but even then, it is important to make sure that the pain is
from the scoliosis and not from some other cause that can
be treated without surgery. Many surgeons are reluctant to

operate on adults with scoliosis because there is a greater risk of complications.

Risks of Surgery

Every surgical procedure carries a risk with it, and spinal fusion surgery is no different. The worst risk, one that every surgeon is required by law to mention to patients, is the possibility of injury to the sensitive spinal cord or nerve roots in the spinal column, and possibly even paralysis. These neurological injuries are rare, occurring in less than 1 percent of scoliosis operations overall. Other complications include infections and failure of the bone to fuse, which is called pseudoarthrosis.

The risk of complications from surgery in adolescents is extremely low, much lower than in adults. Because the bones of adults are no longer developing, they take much longer to heal, even if there are no complications. If surgery is necessary, this is one reason families may decide to have it done while the patient is in her teens.

The possibility of complications, however minimal, is the reason that scoliosis surgery should always be performed by an orthopedic surgeon with extensive experience in this kind of surgery. Scoliosis is a common orthopedic problem for children and teens, and spinal fusion surgery is now a frequently performed operation at many larger hospitals. The Scoliosis Research Society can provide a list of orthopedic surgeons specializing in scoliosis in your area. There are many experienced doctors and hospitals, and selecting a surgeon from among their ranks can help reduce risks to a minimum.

The Cosmetic Debate

When I was a kid, doctors went to great lengths to paint terrible pictures of what would happen if I didn't have surgery. They scared me by saying I wouldn't be able to stand upright, to breathe properly, or to have babies. They said this with great certainty, so that my parents and I would understand the need for surgery. But one thing they never said was, "You will look much better if you have surgery."

Increasingly, physicians and patients are beginning to understand that appearance plays a legitimate role in the decision to have surgery. Even if she could be assured that her health would not be affected in any way, a twelve-year-old girl has every right to be concerned about the prospect of having a severely deformed back as an adult. Although cosmesis should not be the only factor, it should certainly be taken into consideration.

Dr. Thomas Haher told me, "We suddenly realized that we scoliosis specialists, a bunch of middle-aged men, were making decisions for a lot of teenaged girls, and we didn't have the foggiest idea what was important to them."

For some, the word cosmesis conjures up images of elective plastic surgery—women having their noses bobbed or their breasts augmented for no medical reason. But that's not what it means. Very few people choose to have costly, painful, time-consuming scoliosis surgery for purely cosmetic reasons. Legitimate health considerations figure into the decision. On the other hand, although we don't really know what associated health problems will result from a severe spinal curvature in any individual case, we do know that the person will look deformed, and it's a good bet she will have increased back pain.

Surgery will not give you a perfect-looking back. There will be scars, probably long ones. At first, these will be very noticeable in a bathing suit, though they do fade with time. Although the correction with surgery is better than with a brace, 100 percent correction is usually not possible. Still, you will probably stand taller and straighter after surgery. People may tell you what good posture you have. You couldn't slump if you wanted to, because a portion of your spine is now fused. You should tell your surgeons if some aspect of your scoliosis, such as a rib hump, really bothers you, so that the surgeon can choose a specific operative procedure to address that problem.

Dr. Lubicky explained to me why he might recommend observation with the possibility of surgery, rather than bracing, in certain situations: "It's a matter of degree. If a kid comes in, even a very young girl who comes in with a 40-degree curve and has a big rib hump, she's going to look no different after wearing a brace for four years than she does when you start. Her back's not going to look any better, even if the curve never gets a degree bigger. When you present that to patients, especially in a borderline case, they're going to say, 'Why the heck do I want to wear a brace for four or five years if my back's going to look exactly the same?'

"In those situations, I offer patients the option to do nothing. Some of them will say, 'Well, I'll wear the brace, and we'll see what happens.' But I think that when we prescribe things, we have to let patients know what outcome to expect. I think the worst thing you can do is say,

'Oh, we're going to put this brace on, and everything's going to be fine.' To us, if we get to the end of their growth and we stop the brace and we get an X ray five years later and the curve is no bigger than it was the day we put it on, we'll say, 'Hey, this was a success!' Well, the girl still has a big rib hump that she hates, and to her the brace wasn't a success."

Dr. Lubicky stresses that he offers the option of surgery to patients—not that he advocates rushing into surgery. Still, cosmesis is one legitimate consideration.

An Inflexible Problem?

Loss of flexibility is one argument against a spinal fusion. By definition, surgery fuses the spine, transforming it from a collection of movable vertebrae and discs into a solid piece of bone. This is done with the help of "hardware"— rods, hooks, and other items. The fusion does result in some loss of flexibility. There will be activities you may not be able to do as well again, such as gymnastics.

"When patients hear about the stiffness, they say, 'I'll never be able to bend over again.'" Dr. Lubicky told me. "That isn't true. When we bend and sit, we move our hip joints. You're not going to be flexible in the usual sense, but for usual activities that you need to do every day, there really shouldn't be any difference. You might need to do things a little differently. For example, when you need to pick something up, you should do it by squatting down, rather than bending forward."

Having a spinal fusion shouldn't keep you from engaging in most athletic activities, with the possible exception of sports that involve physical contact or a great deal of twisting and bending. Even then, it depends on how experienced you are prior to the fusion. Should the loss of flexibility influence anyone to avoid scoliosis surgery? A professional athlete or dancer would certainly have to consider whether the benefit of surgery would outweigh the risk of spinal stiffness. For most people, however, stiffness alone is not an insurmountable obstacle.

A Painful Decision?

If you have adolescent idiopathic scoliosis, it probably doesn't cause you much pain. It's only fair to warn you that scoliosis surgery is painful, at least at first.

"I didn't expect it to hurt so much," Sara Rubin confessed. Samantha Fish also admitted to a "few days" of severe pain following surgery. Still, all the teens I interviewed felt the surgery was worth the pain and discomfort, especially in view of the possibility that not having surgery might lead to prolonged pain in the future. Also, there are very effective ways of controlling postoperative pain.

Weighing the Options

No outsider can tell you whether to have surgery. It's up to you and your family to weigh all the options and come up with a decision. However, I can tell you what not to do. Don't panic, and don't rush into anything.

Scoliosis is not a medical emergency. Even if you have an advanced curvature, you have time to consider all the treatments available. Your doctor may recommend one treatment over another, perhaps even recommending surgery, but it is ultimately your decision. Take all the time you need before making up your mind. It's important that you and your family:

1. Get a second medical opinion—and a third and a fourth, if necessary, to feel confident that you are making a well-informed decision;

2. Do your homework by learning all you can about scoliosis;

3. Talk it over.

Even if you like and trust your doctor immensely, even if he or she is the person you want to do any surgery should it be necessary, a second medical opinion is a good idea. If a second doctor comes to the same conclusion as the first, both you and the surgeon should feel more confident in the original decision. If the second doctor disagrees, you are perfectly justified in seeking additional opinions before making up your mind.

When my parents and I were considering surgery, our orthopedist had a conference with several other orthopedists on the staff of the hospital. Not surprisingly, they all agreed with him that surgery was necessary. Before my mother would consent, however, she insisted on taking me to a surgeon in another hospital. Not until he said surgery was the way to go did she and my father give their consent.

When looking for a doctor to give a second opinion, try to find a doctor who is as independent as possible. Sometimes this involves a considerable expenditure of time and effort. Your parents have to find the doctor (the Scoliosis Research Society's list is a good place to start), make the appointment, and get your doctor or hospital to release all the necessary records, including X rays, so that the consulting physician can make an informed judgment. Often this means going to a doctor's office or hospital radiology department, signing out the X rays, and carrying them to the second physician's office. If you live in a small community, you may have to travel to another city.

Sounds like a hassle? It is, but when you consider the investment of time, money, and pain involved in major orthopedic surgery, an independent second opinion is worth the time and effort. As for expense, second opinions before major surgery are often required and frequently covered, even if not required, by many health insurance companies.

It's important that you and your family listen carefully to each of the doctors you visit and that you ask plenty of questions so that you understand not only what the surgeon is recommending but why he or she recommends it. When the consulting doctor gives additional reasons for the course of action the first physician recommended, you may feel reassured that the first doctor was right. Or you may prefer the second doctor to the first because his reasons are more compelling.

The next step is homework. If you're reading this book, you are already doing yours, and your parents will probably do some, too. You may want to check out sources on the Internet, the For Further Reading list at the end of this book, or your local library. Look for the most up-to-date publications. The structure of the human spine hasn't changed in centuries, but new surgical techniques are being developed all the time.

If you haven't already done so, this is a good time for you and your parents to join a scoliosis support group. There's no substitute for talking to people who have "been there, done that." Of course, no two people are identical. Hearing why other people did, or did not, choose surgery, may help you to make a more informed decision. After the decision is made—one way or the other—you can continue to seek support from, and give help to, others who are in the same situation. The Scoliosis Association has chapters throughout the United States, but if you can't find a chapter in your area, check with your medical center or physician. Some surgeons or orthopedic departments organize their own scoliosis support groups.

Besides sharing your concerns with others, you may want to share them with yourself. Many teens who keep diaries have found this a good way of dealing with anxieties. Once they're on the paper, they don't gnaw at you quite as much. If you don't keep a diary, you may want to start one, looking forward to the day that you can write, "Well, that's over!" Diary-keeping is not for everyone, but if you enjoy writing, you may find that it helps.

Whatever the final decision, it's very important that you and your parents know each others' feelings. Suppose they decide that you should have surgery and you go along with what they want, but actually you're angry or frightened. You won't be doing yourself, or anyone else, a favor, because your attitude will work against your speedy recovery. On the other hand, your parents may decide against surgery because they want to spare you the pain.

If you feel that pain is a small price to pay for a straighter back, you need to speak out. Communication is important, even if you finally "agree to disagree."

The Cost of Surgery

If your family has agreed on the need for surgery, there may still seem to be some obstacles in your way. What are they and how can you deal with them?

Money would appear to be the most obvious problem. The cost of a complicated operation like a spinal fusion is staggering. Costs may range from as little as $6,000 to as much as $100,000, with figures in the $30,000 range often mentioned. Some factors that influence cost figures are: the geographic location of the hospital, coverage by insurance plans, the specific procedure being performed, the length of the hospital stay, and "extras," such as nursing care or a private room.

Today most insurance companies cover scoliosis surgery. You will want to contact your insurance carrier before having scoliosis surgery. Many insurance policies require policyholders to pay a deductible, which could run to several thousand dollars, after which they cover 80 percent of the remaining costs. If your family belongs to a health maintenance organization (HMO), the HMO may pay the entire cost, but only if you use a surgeon who participates in their plan.

What if you can't pay anything and you don't have insurance? Many hospitals operate clinics that offer free care. Shriners Hospitals for Crippled Children are another choice. They are a network of hospitals that generally treat children free of charge and specialize in orthopedic care. They are excellent hospitals with highly skilled physicians and surgeons. Ask your doctor to refer you if you think that is an option you would like to explore.

There are twenty-two Shriners Hospitals for Crippled Children across North America, nineteen of which are exclusively devoted to pediatric orthopedic care. These hospitals offer state-of-the-art treatment at no cost, with specialists who treat thousands of scoliosis cases each year. New patients are accepted up to age eighteen, with follow-up continuing until the patient is twenty-one years old.

Scoliosis services at these hospitals range from watchful waiting through bracing and surgery. Former patients say there's no better place for a young person to have surgery. The nurses and auxiliary staff are compassionate and caring, and there are plenty of other teens around with whom to share experiences. See the Where to Go for Help section at the end of this book for more information.

The federally funded Medicaid program may also be able to help you. To apply, check with your physician or state agency.

Fitting It In

Scheduling the surgery may pose a problem. First, the doctor you want may not be available at a time convenient to you. Or the doctor may be available for surgery, but may be unavailable during your recovery period. It's important to choose a doctor who is well recommended and who also relates well to you and your family. Try to adjust your schedule to coincide with the doctor's. While you're scheduling, be sure that the doctor will be available for follow-up visits as well.

The doctor's schedule is important, but so is yours. Your parents may decide that surgery is necessary, and while you agree with them, they may want you to have the surgery the week before the big dance or swim meet that you've been anticipating all year. As we've said before, scoliosis is not an emergency. If the doctor's schedule is open, you can schedule the operation when it works best for you. You may want to consider having the surgery during summer vacation so you won't miss too much school.

This doesn't mean you should say, "Yes, I'll have surgery, but not for a year or two, or five," just because it may seem inconvenient. That's procrastinating, and it's only delaying the inevitable. If you have to have surgery, it's much better to have it as a teenager. You'll heal better and faster, and many pediatric orthopedic surgeons won't do follow-up care after you are an adult.

The Moment of Truth

You and your parents have done research, weighed all the options, and talked it over. You may have decided that surgery is advisable, and the sooner the better, or that surgery has to be done, but a few months, or even a year, won't make a big difference. Or you may have decided that you're not going to have surgery. There's no wrong decision, as long as you all come to the conclusion that you're doing the right thing. If you and your parents absolutely can't agree, you may want to ask a trusted friend, counselor, or doctor for an opinion.

If you've decided to postpone surgery, your doctor may

suggest that you continue to wear a brace, to prevent the curve from progressing. Physical therapy and prescribed exercises will help tone your muscles and keep you limber. A bodywork program such as Pilates or Feldenkrais can improve your posture and muscle tone—and your self-confidence. Practicing yoga will help you to stand straighter and feel better physically and mentally.

The thought of having surgery is bound to cause you some anxiety. Some anxiety is not necessarily bad. It can force you to think things through carefully and face your fears. It may help you to acquire as much information as you can to deal with your questions and concerns. Try to develop a support network of friends and family. Try to find others who have undergone surgery, so that you can talk to them. You may also want to ask your doctor about relaxation techniques to help with your anxiety.

If you decide against surgery, and then ten or fifteen years from now you decide you need an operation, is it still an option? What if your curve has progressed significantly, or you have marked back pain which is definitely from the scoliosis? All is not lost. While most surgeons prefer operating on younger patients, many excellent surgeons perform surgery on adults, with excellent outcomes. Carla Podzius had surgery as an adult, as have many others. So whatever the decision, it will probably be the right one.

Surgery—
State of the Art

Michael Buff had a Harrington rod. Sara Rubin had C-D rods, as did Samantha Fish. Alicia Peterman has Paragon instrumentation. I have no hardware.

Harrington rods, C-D rods, and Paragon instrumentation are a few of the different kinds of "hardware" used in scoliosis surgery. They are pieces of metal that are inserted into the spinal area during spinal fusion surgery to help the bone heal into one solid piece and correct the curve. Doctors often combine elements of different hardware systems to achieve the best surgical results.

Surgery is the only method known today of correcting, instead of simply arresting, a spinal curvature. By fusing spinal segments (vertebrae) into a solid piece of bone, surgeons can reduce a curve by many degrees. Of course, as discussed earlier, surgery rarely straightens out the spine completely, but it can correct scoliosis significantly. This correction adds inches to the patient's height, improves appearance, takes pressure off internal organs such as the heart, lungs, and stomach, and frequently enhances the overall quality of life. Patients who have successful scoliosis surgery as teens can discard their braces, engage in most athletic activities, and enjoy life.

Some Basic Principles of Orthopedic Surgery

With the exception of medical professionals, most of us have seen human bones only in skeletons in natural history museums or science class. So we may not realize bones are living tissue like skin or muscle. Because bones are living tissue, new bone cells can form. This enables bones to heal after trauma or surgery into a new, stronger bone, making successful scoliosis surgery possible.

Before I go into detail about scoliosis surgery, it may be helpful to think about what happens when someone breaks a bone. If the break is a simple fracture, meaning the bone is cracked but hasn't shifted position, the arm or leg is put in a cast or brace until it heals. If the bone is cracked and dislocated (has shifted out of alignment), the break is called a compound fracture. The doctor will try to reset the bones of a compound fracture, forcing the bones back into alignment by applying pressure from outside. The doctor will then put the leg or arm in a cast. If this is not enough to hold the reset bones in place, a surgeon will put the pieces of bone back together and use hardware (metal screws or pins) to hold the reset bones in place while they heal.

The spine is not one solid bone but a collection of vertebrae, each of which is hollow in the center. The nerves of the spinal cord run through this series of hollow centers, which together form the spinal canal. For this reason spinal surgery is more complicated than setting an arm or leg, but the same principles apply. To fuse a portion of the spine into a solid piece, the surgeon removes material from between the vertebrae, places the vertebrae in the correct position—often using a metal rod or hardware "system" to align it—and then grafts bone from elsewhere in the patient's body to help the bone fuse. The hardware remains in the body during the healing process to support the spine and promote fusion.

Your surgeon will decide how long to make the fusion and what kind of hardware to use, taking into account the type, size, and location of the curve. A double major curve may require a more extensive fusion than a short thoracic or lumbar curve. If the fusion is too long, the spine may lose too much flexibility. If it's too short, the fusion may not hold. The doctor will aim for the best possible correction with the least possible loss of flexibility. His or her skill, and the use of increasingly sophisticated hardware, help achieve this goal.

In the last chapter, you learned that the neck ring of the Milwaukee brace was designed to pull on the top of the spine, while the pads of the brace pushed on the curve. Metal rods and hooks perform a similar function, with the hooks pulling and the rod pushing. Some hardware can also help reduce a rib hump by "derotating" vertebrae that have rotated away from the midline.

A Brief History

When I had surgery, the surgeon grafted bone from my hip to my spine, to fill up the space between the vertebrae and hold the spine in a straighter position. Because the doctors could fuse only a few vertebrae at a time, they had to operate twice—once on the upper curve and once on the lower. I had to be kept immobile to allow the fusion to heal, so I was in a body cast in bed for three months afterward and a walking cast for another two months after that. I had to stay in the hospital all summer. The walking cast prevented me from taking a bath or shower for another two months. However, I did heal, and the operation was a success.

Michael Buff had surgery in 1980, long after the invention of the first "hardware"—the Harrington rod. He was in the hospital for only two weeks, though he had to wear a walking cast for six months. Michael would have liked to take a real bath, but he was not sorry that the cast kept him from wearing a suit and tie—the standard dress code for his school—and, thanks to the Harrington rod, he was quite mobile and didn't have to miss school.

Harrington Rod

The Harrington rod technique was developed by Dr. Paul Harrington of Houston, Texas, in the 1940s. When a Harrington rod is used, hooks are attached to the vertebrae at each end of the curve. A thin metal rod with notches is passed through them. The rod works on the principle of distraction, forcing the two ends of the curve farther apart. After the hooks and rod are in place, the surgeon gently moves the top hook up the notched rod, lifting up the vertebra at the top of the curve and thus helping to pull the spine straight. It is much like the way a mechanic lifts a car up on a jack. Although most Harrington rod patients wore walking casts, the rod did allow them to move around during their recovery. Most people who have surgery today are up and around in a few days. They don't even have to wear a brace after surgery.

The Harrington rod system was a great stride forward in scoliosis surgery, although today, the original Harrington rods are used by only about 2 percent of scoliosis surgeons. Some modified versions, such as the Drummond system, are also still in use. One drawback of the original Harrington rod was that, because it was attached only at the top and bottom of the curve, it was possible for it to break in the middle. Although it certainly wasn't common, this did happen with some of the early Harrington rods. The improved versions, such as the Drummond system, seldom break.

Segmental Systems

Today, most surgeons use some type of segmental system. This means the hardware is fixed to the spine at a number of points, so that there is less stress on the ends. The first segmental system was the Cotrel-Dubousset system—the "C-D rods" worn by Samantha and Sara—introduced in the 1980s. Alicia's Paragon instrumentation is another variety, as are TSRH (Texas Scottish Rite Hospital), Isola, and Miami-Moss.

In addition to distraction, or forcing the two ends of the curve farther apart, segmental systems use two additional methods of correcting a curve. Through rod rotation, surgeons can "derotate" a curve to some extent, decreasing the patient's kyphosis or "humpback." By using a segmental system, the surgeon can also pull the curve closer, but not all the way, to the midline. In other words, he can make a big C into a gently bending line, like a parenthesis (.

Many doctors feel the segmental systems are better than the old rods because they provide more stabilization, greater correction, better balance, and higher rates of successful fusion. Doctors are also able to contour the rods of the segmental systems to help keep the normal front-to-back curve intact. In the early days of spinal instrumentation, patients often came out of surgery with a condition called "flatback," which resulted in lower back pain. Today, surgeons are much more careful about preserving the normal front-to-back curve. Segmental systems cut down or eliminated the need for casts or braces after surgery and vastly decreased the amount of time patients needed to remain immobile, either in the hospital or at home.

C-D Systems, Zielke System, and Luque Instrumentation

When I visited his laboratory, Steve Caruso at St. Vincent's Medical Center showed me two plaster and metal models. One of these was a Cotrel-Dubousset system. The C-D system is a vast improvement over the Harrington rod system. But, Steve explained, "the difficulty with the C-D system is that it is a global correction. Hooks are placed far apart. You have stresses and forces at the hooks, and they are not distributed evenly along the curve." This leads to a relatively long, stiff fusion, with stress above and below.

The other model was of a Zielke system. It was much smaller than the C-D rods and involved fewer vertebrae. "This is a very thin rod," Steve said. "What this allows you to do is to segmentally distribute the stresses you are applying along the curve." Because the Zielke rod is thin, patients do have to wear a brace for a time after surgery (but not a cast—so they can bathe). Some doctors believe the advantages of a shorter fusion and a thinner rod may be more comfort in the long run, outweighing the disadvantage of the cast. This system is not widely used today, but some doctors find it useful for certain fusions.

Another system, Luque (pronounced LOO-key) instrumentation, uses two rods attached to the vertebrae by thin wires, called sublaminar wires. Because the wires go into the spinal canal, possibly increasing the risk of nerve damage, Luque is also used infrequently. Michelle Ann Mauney's surgeons used Luque instrumentation successfully in her surgery.

Leaving Hardware In

Most patients are never conscious of the hardware used to correct scoliosis once it has been surgically attached, but some are. This is more often true of the hooks than the rods, because there are more hooks, and they are nearer your skin. If a hook really bothers you, you can ask to have it out after a year or so, when the bone has fused. The job of the hardware is to support the spine while the bone fuses. It provides internal fixation and either eliminates or reduces the need for a cast or brace. After a year or more, fusion should have taken place and you can have the hardware removed if you like. If the hardware doesn't bother you, you'll probably decide to leave it in rather than have major surgery a second time.

These are examples of a few hardware systems. Your surgeon may combine elements of several systems or may

133

use another system altogether. The important thing is to pick a surgeon you trust.

Getting Ready for Surgery

If you are already physically active, especially if you participate in a physical fitness program two or three times a week—either in school or outside—that's great. If you haven't been active outside of your weekly gym class, try to increase your activities. Either way, be sure that a good part of your workout is aerobic, aimed at increasing your heart rate and lung capacity. Your lungs need to be in good shape for the anesthesia. Taking part in an exercise, aerobic dance, or swimming program is good for your mental outlook as well. It gives you a chance to make new friends or to work out with old ones, and it makes you feel good about yourself. Also, the physical therapist who is part of the scoliosis team at your medical center may give you exercises to keep you limber and improve your breathing.

In the weeks before your surgery, the doctor may order new spinal X rays to get an up-to-date picture of your scoliosis. He or she may also ask you to see your pediatrician or internist for a thorough checkup, just to make sure there are no other health problems. You'll need blood transfusions during surgery, and you may be asked to donate your own blood in advance for this purpose. You can't donate the week of surgery, so your weekly donations will start well in advance. Giving your own blood (autologous donation) is a safeguard against blood-borne infections.

If you want to talk to someone who's had surgery, ask

your doctor. Many scoliosis surgeons have the names of former patients who will be happy to talk with you on the phone. Your local Scoliosis Association also may be able to put you in touch with someone who's been through the experience. The important thing is not where you get the help from, but that you get it.

Before Your Surgery

In the week before surgery, you'll go to the hospital for preadmission testing. These tests are required even if you've had a general checkup in the past six months. They include blood tests, urine analysis, sometimes a chest X ray, and a general physical. While you're there, you and your parents may meet with the anesthesiologist, who will keep you asleep during the surgery. He or she will ask about your medical history to determine what anesthesia is right for you, and you'll get a chance to ask questions. Most pediatric units in hospitals will also give you a short tour so that you can see where you'll be recuperating.

You won't need to pack much to take to the hospital, but you may want to take out your suitcase several days before, so that you can put things in as you think of them. Avoid bringing money or other valuables. Take along some comfortable pajamas (although for a few days after surgery, you will have to wear a hospital gown), a nightgown or bathrobe, and perhaps something with sentimental value, such as a favorite stuffed animal or a good-luck charm. Foot coverings—socks to keep your feet warm and slippers to walk in—are necessary.

You may not feel like reading much and you probably

won't do any schoolwork in the hospital, but take a favorite book or some quiet games. Your parents may visit you a lot. Some hospitals allow a parent to stay overnight. So even if you don't feel like reading, Mom or Dad may be happy to read to you or play a game or two. There will be a television in your room, but you may want to bring an inexpensive personal stereo and some tapes or CDs you like, so that you can choose your own music.

The day before your surgery, you'll have a million details to take care of. But the day before that might be a good time to try to relax and take your mind off the operation. My surgery took place in New York City, 130 miles away from home, so my mother treated me to a night in a hotel, lunch, and a movie before we had to check into the hospital. It was a "girls' day out" I never forgot. If possible, you and your family can think about planning some fun activity, or just have a sleep-over or a lunch date with a good friend to get you in a mellow mood.

At the Hospital

The procedures governing how long before surgery patients have to check into the hospital may vary according to the hospital rules, the doctor's preference, and your insurance coverage. At Chicago Shriners Hospital, patients are admitted no later than one day before surgery. At other hospitals, patient registration and discussion with the anesthesiologist are done during the preadmission testing, and patients are told to report to the surgical unit on the day of surgery. So although some of the procedures I've described may take place in a different sequence, they will still take place at some point prior to surgery.

You won't be allowed any food or water for at least eight hours before the operation. If you're already checked in at the hospital, the order "Nothing by mouth after midnight" will be written on your chart. If you're at home, the doctor will give you and your parents instructions that you are not to eat or even drink water after midnight. This is done to reduce the likelihood of nausea and vomiting when you are given an anesthetic.

After you have checked into the hospital and been given a room, you may be visited by members of the team who will be doing your surgery and postoperative care. Nurses may stop by to tell you what your recovery time will be like, someone from anesthesiology may run a final check on you, and a physical therapist may also stop by to talk about how he or she will be helping you after surgery.

The Day of Surgery

Even if you are nervous the day before surgery, the chances are you won't feel as nervous the day of surgery. You may sleep restlessly and wake early, but you'll find plenty of people to answer any last-minute questions and keep you calm and reassured. You'll also be busy getting ready. If you arrive at the hospital on the day of surgery, there will be a brief admitting procedure, although most of the formalities will probably have been taken care of in preadmission. All patients then change into hospital gowns and are put in bed to be "prepped" for surgery. Usually, your parents can stay with you through most of the preparation. In some cases, they will even be allowed to walk alongside your gurney (wheeled stretcher) as far as the operating room doors.

During the prep period, you'll be hooked up to IV (intravenous, or into-the-vein) equipment. An IV allows necessary fluids to flow into you during surgery. A small needle is inserted into your arm, usually at the inside of your elbow and a plastic tube runs from the needle to a bag hanging on a nearby stand. The fluids may be antibiotics, blood, saline solution, or anything else that the doctor knows you will need during surgery. The IV may be kept in your arm for a day or two after the operation.

Exactly when patients are given anesthesia differs from hospital to hospital and from doctor to doctor, but it's a sure bet that you won't remember anything about the surgery. Sometimes patients are given something to relax them while they are still in their room, and they are wheeled into the operating room in a pleasant haze. Other times the anesthesiologist administers the anesthesia in the operating room itself. In any case, you'll be anesthetized before the surgery starts.

Waking Up

"When I woke up, I was in the recovery room. I didn't know what was going on," said Samantha Fish. "I didn't feel any pain yet, but everything felt so distant."

"I woke up with a tube down my throat," said Alicia Peterman. "I couldn't move my feet because of the anesthetic. I thought I was paralyzed."

"I didn't expect it to hurt so much," Sara Rubin said.

The first few days after any surgery are not easy, and sco-liosis surgery is no exception. Pain and disorientation are to be expected. That's the downside. The upside is that, complicated as it sounds to you and me, scoliosis surgery is a common procedure for the surgical teams that per-form it routinely. It's all part of a day's work to them, and most are incredibly good at it.

Procedures vary at different hospitals, but you'll be kept either in the recovery room or the intensive care unit (ICU) for a while after surgery. You will probably also find yourself hooked to many machines that monitor your health.

In addition to the IV that was attached before surgery, there may be a second IV to give you blood. If you donated blood in advance, this will be the time when your own blood comes back to you, to replace what you lost during surgery. One of the IVs may also be con-nected to a patient controlled analgesia (PCA) pump, which administers pain medication in safe doses. It may be controlled by the patient or set up to give a continu-ous dose. Samantha Fish was allowed to control her PCA pump, and she felt that it helped lessen her postopera-tive pain.

You may wake up with an incredible urge to urinate. This is because a Foley catheter—a small rubber tube—has been inserted into the opening through which you uri-nate. This tube, connected to a collection bag, allows the nurses to measure your urine output. It makes you feel like you have to go, when you are actually "going" and don't know it. However, this feeling will soon pass.

If you watch doctor shows on television, you have

seen people in the recovery room with tubes in their noses. Patients coming out of surgery are routinely connected to an oxygen supply for a day or two, either with tubes or an oxygen mask, so that their lungs are well ventilated.

At the site of the incision, there will be a small plastic tube connected to a container called a Hemovac, which drains the wound of excess blood and fluid. Hemovacs are used in a number of surgical procedures. You'll have to put up with it for a while when you're in the hospital, but it's no big deal.

If your surgery was the kind that was close to the lungs or stomach, a tube may be inserted into your chest cavity and connected to a small drainage container. This equipment helps keep the lungs inflated and prevents blood and fluid from accumulating in the chest. You may also have a nasogastric (nose-to-stomach) tube inserted to keep your stomach empty after surgery. These tubes are a nuisance, but they will probably be taken out before you leave the recovery room or ICU.

There's one more technical term that is useful to know: log-rolling. Usually scoliosis patients wake up from surgery lying on their backs. Since they are not able to move very much, nurses roll them from their backs to their sides every two or three hours to prevent bedsores, which develop if you lie too long in one position.

No one is hungry after major surgery like a spinal fusion, but you may be very thirsty. For a day or two, the IV will give you all the nutrition you're going to get, but a wet cloth on your lips or a few ice chips held in your mouth may help to slake your thirst.

It Only Hurts When I Laugh

Whether you're like Sara, who "didn't expect it to hurt so much," or Samantha, who didn't feel any pain when she woke up, there will be a good deal of pain in the days immediately following your surgery. Sometimes the pain doesn't really hit until a day or so after the operation, because you will probably be on heavy pain medication. If you have a PCA pump, you'll be allowed to control your own dosage of pain medication, within reason, and this does help. The PCA pump will be discontinued after the first few days, and the doctor will prescribe a painkiller that can be taken orally. You may be given a prescription you can fill after you get home, or the doctor will suggest an over-the-counter painkiller, such as Tylenol. After a while, you shouldn't need anything, but if something really hurts, you should tell the doctor.

Of course, the pain doesn't disappear immediately, but it does go away gradually. As you start being more active and getting back into your routine, you may have a temporary increase in pain, but that is to be expected. Codeine and some other narcotic medications make you constipated, and that may make you feel worse than the actual pain. Tell your doctor; he or she will either change your pain medication or give you something for the constipation.

Don't be surprised if your worst pain comes from unlikely places. If you've had bone removed for a graft, the incision where the bone was removed may hurt more than the graft itself. Or the muscles that were shoved aside to get at the bone may complain.

You're not going to feel better every day than you did the day before. Some days will be worse than others. But you will feel better over time. The teens I spoke to all felt a good deal better in a week, much better in a month, and "all better" a year after surgery.

The Road to Recovery

Dr. Areta Podhorodecki is a physiatrist—a physician who specializes in rehabilitation medicine. She is part of the team that treats scoliosis patients at St. Vincent's Medical Center in New York City. She is actively involved with surgical patients, as well as some patients with scoliosis who do not have surgery.

"The physiatrist is the leader of the rehabilitation team," Dr. Podhorodecki explained. "We know what rehab can do for patients. With a team you can delegate and designate, whether it be physical and occupational therapy or speech therapy. With scoliosis, we write the prescription for physical therapy, for the therapist to treat a patient and design an exercise protocol.

"When a patient has surgery, the whole rehab team is involved," she continued. "I see patients even when they are still in intensive care. After surgery, we get them up right away. Immediately after surgery, we get them moving their lungs so that they won't get pneumonia. Often we get them from the bed to a chair and try a few steps without a brace."

The process of rehabilitation begins as soon as you come back from the recovery room or intensive care. Unlike in the recovery room, where you are more or less helpless and everything is done for you, you must be an active participant in your own rehabilitation. This means following doctor's orders. The phrase "for your own good" is never more appropriate than in the days right after surgery. If the doctor, nurse, or therapist tells you to get out of bed or walk a few steps, you have to do it, whether or not it hurts. The more you do it, the easier it gets. That doesn't mean you should try to do more than you're told. Physiatrists and physical therapists have worked with hundreds, maybe thousands, of patients. They know what kind of activity, and how much, is appropriate at each stage of your recovery.

"After a few days, the therapist comes in," Samantha says. "They try and make you walk to the end of the bed and sit down. Then they make you walk to the end of the room. You can't leave the hospital until you can walk up and down stairs."

"The physiatrist is the liaison between the surgeon and the rest of the team. The surgeon is usually very occupied with surgery, very busy in the operating room all day," Dr. Podhorodecki explained. "The rehab doctor is interested in function. The physiatrist stresses independence in living, activities of daily living, and self-care. This is supervised learning. Rehab is nice because people feel they can test themselves with somebody watching them, and if they hurt themselves you can address it immediately. And if they don't hurt themselves, they can see how far they can go, and they feel very reassured about that. That's very important in low back pain, especially with people returning to work [or school]."

When Can I Get Out of Here?

The big difference between scoliosis surgery today and when I had my operation is the length of the hospital stay and the degree of immobilization. I was in the hospital for three months in a cast that reached from my neck to the top of my legs. Today, hospital stays are generally around a week—six to eight days, to be exact.

Doctors do put their patients in braces after surgery when necessary, but this is more true for adults than for children and teens. The hardware inside the spine provides support, frequently making postoperative braces or casts unnecessary. Dr. Lubicky told me that the Milwaukee brace still comes in handy for patients who need extra support after surgery. Dr. Haher says he often gives the patient a brace when he uses Zielke instrumentation, because the rods are quite thin.

Whether or not you have to wear a brace, you'll be out of the hospital soon. Looking back, you'll be amazed at how much progress you made within a few days. When you first come to your room from the recovery room or intensive care, you may still have some of the tubes and other impediments to normal functioning I have described. Within a few days, all of these will be removed. You'll probably go from IV to Jell-O and soft foods to normal food. Don't be surprised if your appetite is not wonderful for a while—you've been through major surgery; you're not physically active; and hospital food is usually pretty boring. Besides, the medication you're taking may upset your stomach.

Most orthopedic units where pediatric scoliosis surgery

is performed are excellent at responding to both the physical and psychological needs of children and teens. The nurses and other staff members are highly trained and sensitive to patients' concerns. In many cases, you'll have roommates to keep you company and share your feelings. Also, parents can either sleep over or, at the very least, visit frequently.

Still, you shouldn't be surprised if you don't feel like your cheerful self the whole time you're in the hospital. Hospitals aren't easy to get used to: People wake you up early and bring your breakfast late. They are constantly asking you questions or poking around your body; and then, when you want someone, it seems like forever until they answer your call. Also, it's natural for your moods to fluctuate during recovery. Your first reaction may be, "I'm glad that's over," but after you've checked that all your arms and legs are basically in working order, you start to get restless. You wish that the whole process was over— not just the surgery.

If you feel "blue" from time to time, that's normal. Your mood will gradually get better, with little dips of self-pity, until one day you realize that you're back to normal. When Samantha Fish told me, "Everything's perfect," she really sounded on top of the world.

In the next chapter, we'll talk more about what happens when you get home.

The First Day of the Rest of Your Life

A fourteen-year-old girl named Maria had scoliosis surgery. Before surgery she had a 45-degree curve. The surgery reduced it to less than 10 degrees. One of her ribs was removed. The surgeon fused five vertebrae and inserted a stainless steel rod. A tube was inserted into her lungs, which allowed for drainage. Three days later, the tube was removed. After the surgery, she was given an oral painkiller.

Five days after the surgery, Maria was released from the hospital a day early, because her doctor felt her recovery was proceeding more quickly than usual. As a result of surgery, Maria gained about one and a half inches in height, as predicted.

A week after surgery, Maria was feeling so good that she didn't rest enough, and the next day her pain increased. She rested and felt better. She felt so good that her parents had to keep reminding her not to try to do too much in the first several days after surgery. Maria continued to take medication to control the pain, but much less frequently.

The one reason for having scoliosis surgery as a preteen or teenager, as opposed to waiting until you are older, is the difference in recovery time. That doesn't mean teens don't have any pain. The story above shows that they do. And there are limitations. Your doctor may place restrictions on the type and amount of physical activity that you can do, at least for a while. Still, generally speaking, no adult would feel as healthy as quickly as would a teenager following major surgery.

Samantha came home from the hospital on a Thursday and went to the movies on Saturday. She was back in school after two and a half weeks. Sara was in the hospital for six days and had to stay home for three weeks. After a month, she could ride her bike. After one month of home tutoring, Alicia went back to school.

There Were Some Changes Made

The most obvious improvement after scoliosis surgery is correction of the spinal curve. Sara's curve went from 50 degrees to 25. Whatever the numbers, many teens experience a strange sensation when they look in the mirror and see their new bodies standing so much straighter and taller. It's not uncommon to gain a few inches in height.

Most people are delighted at the results of their surgery. In the first place, they're happy to be finished with the ordeal. Second, they are happy that they look more "normal" than they did before.

Setting the Pace

Most of the teens I spoke with were glad that they had the surgery and realistic about the fact that some curvature remained. Because I spoke to them quite a while after surgery—anywhere from five months to several years— the memory of the pain and physical limitations had receded to the dim, distant past.

But after surgery there will be pain, and there will be mood swings. Recuperation is an up-and-down process; you go forward three steps and back one. When you come home from the hospital, you may not feel like doing much, or you may feel restless and want to do things but still find that any attempt at activity results in pain and fatigue.

Take it slowly. Set simple goals for yourself each day, such as, "Today, I am going to walk around the room ten times," or "Today, I am going to walk around the block." Walking is very important. You won't be able to walk for more than a few minutes at a time at first—just around your room or to the bathroom. That's normal. At first, you'll need to take a lot of little walks, with big rest periods in between, but as time goes by, the ratio of walking to resting will change. Your doctor may advise you to walk for at least thirty minutes a day.

Even though preteens and teenagers heal much faster than adults, you may have pain when you walk or try new activities. It's normal to say to yourself, "I've just been through major surgery. I'm entitled to be good to myself. I think I'll just sit around the house and watch television."

While it's not good to overdo physical activity following major surgery, it's also important to resist the urge to be inactive during your recovery. Walking strengthens muscles, helps keep you from getting stiff, and helps you to get back to normal faster. Listen to your body and don't do too much at once, but also try not to sit still for more than thirty or forty-five minutes at a time. If you are taking time off to watch a favorite television program, that's okay. Just remember to get up during commercials and walk around, and when the show is over, go take a walk.

Reward yourself for making an effort. Instead of just taking a walk, walk someplace, such as a store or an ice cream parlor. Or take the walk with a good friend, and have a visit at the same time.

In addition to walking, your doctor may tell you to add some low-impact aerobic activities as soon as your wounds have healed. This could be walking on a treadmill or using a stair-climber, skiing machine, or exercise bicycle. Once the incision is completely healed, swimming is an excellent exercise.

Physical Therapy

After your scoliosis surgery, your doctor will probably prescribe physical therapy. Exercises prescribed to help compensate for scoliosis may also help avoid or alleviate lower back pain, now and later.

Physical therapy is tailored to meet your specific needs. It is important that your physical therapist supervise your program because some exercises and treatments may be worthless to you or even cause you harm. The physical therapist will show you the best exercises for your specific type of scoliosis.

The therapist will teach you how to do exercises that will improve your posture, strengthen your back and stomach muscles, and correct imbalances (for example, strengthen muscles that are weaker on one side). If you have pain, the therapist may treat sore muscles with heat, ice, or ultrasound before you exercise. By reducing the pain, this treatment helps you move more freely and exercise better.

I saw a physical therapist for my lower back pain—the result of scoliosis plus normal wear and tear. She applied wet heat and used gentle massage to relax my sore muscles. Then, although I had already been doing some back exercises, she showed me how to perform them more effectively. I still do the exercises every day, plus some yoga. In addition, I go to the gym several times a week for an aerobic workout (mainly walking on a treadmill). It really helps.

The aim of physical therapy is to teach you exercises that you can eventually do at home. The therapist supports and supervises you so that you can't hurt yourself while you are learning. If you like your therapist and he or she works well with you and your treatment team, you are more likely to trust your therapist and successfully complete the prescribed treatment program. If you have a doctor's prescription for the therapy, it will almost certainly be covered by medical insurance.

While specific exercises vary from patient to patient, the goals are basically the same. Scoliosis exercises are designed to:

1. Strengthen the abdominal and trunk extensor muscles;

2. Stretch tight muscles on the concave (indented) side of the curve;

3. Strengthen the lateral trunk flexors (muscles that

help you bend sideways) on the convex (bulging) side of the curve;

4. Stretch tight muscles associated with an increased lumbar lordosis (swayback);

5. Improve your posture.

In some of these exercises, the therapist will physically support you. Other exercises are done by the patient alone, but under the supervision of the therapist. These can be performed on a mat or standing against a wall.

The main reason to see a physiatrist or physical therapist is to have a program tailored to your specific needs and to learn how to do the exercises under supervision, so that you will do a maximum of good and a minimum of harm. After a while, you won't need supervision anymore. The physical therapist will give you a program of exercises, which you will have now learned, to do at home. Even after you are back at school, try to do these exercises every day. They will help improve muscle strength and flexibility and prevent back pain.

An Exercise Timetable

Francesca Halter was diagnosed with scoliosis at age eleven during a school screening. She wore a brace for two years, but her curve continued to increase, so when Francesca was thirteen she had an anterior fusion with Zielke instrumentation. Francesca has never regretted having surgery. "The scars aren't fun, but I do every activity possible," she says.

Prior to her surgery, Francesca was an avid horseback

rider. "My doctor prohibited me from riding for a year. But after a year, I was back in it—a little sore, but it got better. The doctor wouldn't let me dive for a year, either." Here is the schedule of physical activity her doctor gave her.

Three weeks: Walking, light swimming, some stretches

Six weeks: Comfortable light exercise (stationary bicycle, swimming, more stretches)

Three months: Some low-impact exercise (light jogging, Stairmaster)

Six months: Low-impact aerobic exercise (not high-impact; running is okay)

Nine months: Most high-impact aerobics

One year: Diving and horseback riding

This is only one example of a schedule. Yours may be different, and it will depend on your doctor, your body, and the hardware that your doctor uses. Most of the teens I interviewed who had surgery said their doctors asked them to wait a year before engaging in contact sports or other strenuous activity. Most exercise timetables begin with walking, then light activity such as swimming is added. Exercise gradually increases to include low-impact aerobics and finally graduates to high-impact aerobics and sports. Eventually you will be able to return to your presurgical level of activities.

The Future for Backs

What does the future hold for you, a teen with scoliosis? If you did have surgery, does that mean you never have to think about scoliosis again? If you didn't have surgery, will you have problems later? The answer to all three questions is that we don't really know. But that's not bad news; it just means you may have to make some choices later in life.

Suzette Haden Elgin had polio when she was nine, and it left her with scoliosis. Despite doctors' dire predictions that she would be unable to function normally or have children unless she had surgery, Suzette and her family decided not to go that route. Instead, they found a doctor who observed her through her teens and predicted the curve would stabilize once she reached her growth.

"He was wrong," Suzette says. "There was slow but steady progression, all my life. I have had a normal life and have borne four children, despite the predictions. I have a double curve and have no idea about the degrees of either curve, just that they're severe. All this was long ago, of course, and is not relevant today, except to let you know that even doctors' predictions do not always come true."

Whatever you do, try to stay fit. The best thing you can do for yourself is eat right and exercise. If you haven't tried any of the programs I described, such as Feldenkrais, Pilates, or yoga, you still have plenty of time to try them.

If you've had a spinal fusion, it's a good idea to find out which vertebrae were fused and to have the information noted in your medical records for future reference. It is difficult, if not impossible, to get a hypodermic needle into a fused spine. It's not a major problem, but hospital personnel should know about it. If you carry a MedicAlert card, this information should be included. A spinal fusion may prevent a pregnant woman from having a "spinal" or "epidural"—anesthetic administered by means of an injection in the spinal canal—when she gives birth.

Doctors do believe that thoracic curves, if allowed to progress, can interfere with heart and lung functioning later in life. However, this doesn't happen in every case, and the curve must be extremely severe, with a great deal of rotation, before heart or lung functioning is really impeded.

There's no doubt that more research is needed in many areas. First, we need to find out what causes idiopathic scoliosis. If, as many suspect, it is a neurological problem, it is conceivable that a method may be found, many years in the future, to correct the "righting system" in the brain or spinal cord.

Although current surgical procedures have produced excellent short-term results, research is needed in this area. The instrumentation systems currently in use have not been around many years. We will have to wait until girls like Alicia, Sara, and Samantha are in their forties or fifties to find out how well the various types of instrumentation systems function and whether the girls' scoliosis continues to progress. By carefully tracking these current patients, surgeons can continue to refine their techniques.

Regardless of what future research may tell us, we can predict fairly confidently that the vast majority of preteens and teens who are diagnosed with scoliosis today will have few or no future problems. This applies to most people who have mild scoliosis (under 20 degrees) or whose curves have been arrested—by nature, a brace, or surgery—at around 30 degrees.

The problem with predictions like this is that they are based on the law of averages. We can say what happens "in most" or "in the vast majority" of cases, but we can't predict with absolute certainty what will happen to any one specific person. You could be the one person in thousands whose 10-degree curve at age sixteen becomes a 50-degree curve when you are thirty. Or you could have a 60-degree curve at age twenty and still have the same degree of scoliosis thirty years later. It's not probable, but anything is possible.

So what should you do? Do what seems best now and try not to worry. Stay fit; don't become overweight, because that puts a strain on your back. Eat right, because you need nutrients for healthy bones and muscles. Otherwise, the chances are good that, if your curve is either mild or under control, you won't have any problems after you reach skeletal maturity.

Surgery Again?

If you are one of the comparatively few who do require surgery, is there any possibility you may need future surgery? I can't say no, because I've already told the story of Samantha Fish, who had surgery twice—once to correct a pressing problem and once to extend the fusion because she had grown. Also, Francesca Halter, who likes diving and horseback riding, has recently had additional surgery. Her first operation, which was performed when she was thirteen, left her with a "flatback"—an insufficient sagittal (front-to-back, S-shaped) curve. At age twenty, Francesca had additional surgery to correct this condition. Francesca's surgeon said that flatback is not uncommon and that it is related to the degree of the original curve. The early Harrington rods often produced this condition. With newer hardware and more awareness of this possible complication, scoliosis surgeons now try harder to keep the patient's sagittal curve normal.

A second surgery may also be recommended to remove hardware. If a rod breaks, or if the bone fails to fuse, the surgeon may have to operate again. In the early days of scoliosis instrumentation, rods broke more frequently than they do today. As hardware gets better and better, the chances of this kind of complication decrease.

Surgery Later?

Suppose you didn't have surgery as a teen. Is there any reason you might have it later? I can think of several:

1. The curve may progress. While there's no way to predict whether a specific person's scoliosis will progress and by how much, we do know that in general, the greater the curve, the more chance

there is that it will get worse. Most surgeons agree that curves under 30 degrees won't increase after skeletal maturity, and few recommend surgery on teens whose curves are under 40. So could a curve stabilized at 40 or even 45 degrees get worse after full bone growth? Yes, it could. On the other hand, it very well might not. The reason most surgeons strongly recommend surgery for curves over 50 degrees is that those curves probably will get worse if left untreated.

2. Adult scoliosis may develop. Throughout this book, I've said most scoliosis is of the adolescent idiopathic variety. But scoliosis does appear in adults who never knew they had it before. Sometimes they didn't have it, and sometimes it just went undetected. Or it could be degenerative scoliosis, which develops in adults (usually adult women) as a result of the aging process.

3. The scoliosis may become painful. Even if the scoliosis doesn't progress much in terms of degrees, you may decide to have surgery because of pain. Teens with scoliosis don't usually have pain, but adults do, and it is the most common reason for them to have spinal fusions. As you grow older, you become less flexible. If you have an imbalance as a result of scoliosis, you are going to feel it more. This is one excellent reason to stay in shape. Exercise may reduce pain and increase mobility. Also, physical therapy may help. Still, if

your vertebrae are not sitting squarely on top of each other, the discs in between may be affected, and that hurts. During a fusion, the diseased discs are removed and the bone is made into one solid piece. This results in a loss of mobility, but it may reduce the pain. At present, many surgeons are reluctant to perform a fusion if a patient's only symptom is pain, and will do it only as a last resort.

4. Technology may improve. Even if you and your family decide against scoliosis surgery now, who knows what the future may bring? Some surgeons are already using the technique of endoscopy, the use of a lighted telescope called an endoscope, and a video monitor, for certain cases of spinal fusion surgery. This technique is known as video-assisted thorascopy. Surgeons perform anterior (front) scoliosis surgery through the chest cavity (thorax) with the aid of an instrument called a thorascope. The approach requires much smaller incisions than traditional anterior scoliosis surgery, so the recuperation time is much shorter. This is just one example of the kind of technological advances we can expect.

Looking Ahead

In Chapter 5, I said I was not teased after my scoliosis surgery, because of the efforts of my family, friends, and teachers. But there was another reason I was not teased: my own attitude.

Surgery did more than correct my scoliosis. I came back to school with the knowledge that I had confronted a major challenge and triumphed. Throughout my hospital stay, friends and family complimented me for my courage and good humor. Sure, I was afraid. But I had a terrific support network, and I soon realized a positive attitude paid off. People enjoyed visiting me, and I enjoyed their visits. The experience gave me confidence and made me realize that despite what some kids at school might think, I wasn't such a "crybaby" after all.

Of course, it wasn't all smooth sailing from that point forward. Being rejected by the girls I thought were my friends during my first year at college was a bitter blow. But with Jane's help I dealt with that problem, just as I had dealt with scoliosis.

Growing up involves meeting challenges, and scoliosis may be one of them. I hope this book can make coping with scoliosis a learning experience. You've learned what scoliosis is—a lateral curvature of the spine that affects one in every ten teens. You also know what it is not: It's not a disease, and it is almost never an emergency. You and your parents have time to make treatment decisions. If you choose an option such as watchful waiting or bracing, you can still change your mind later. Your participation in the decision-making process can be a positive experience for everyone involved.

Scoliosis teaches teens to "go with the flow." Most kids who wear braces get used to them quickly. They soon ignore the thoughtless remarks of a few insensitive people. They know who their real friends are and avoid those who are too narrow to look beyond the surface and see

see the real person inside. Like Carla, they make new friends and develop new interests.

The best thing about wearing a brace or having surgery for scoliosis is that it doesn't last forever. It's like the joke about the man who said, "I love to hit my head with a hammer. It feels so good when I stop." The brace comes off, the surgery fades into the past. One day, you wake up and realize you haven't thought about your scoliosis for a week, or a month, or even a year. You met the challenge. Other things become much more important—school, athletic activities, dating, a career. Other than an occasional checkup, scoliosis rarely crosses your mind.

But that's the future. Now you or someone you know may be dealing with scoliosis. Or you may have dealt with your own scoliosis and want to use your experience to help others. What can you do?

> **Help others with scoliosis**. If a support group helped you deal with feelings and make treatment decisions, you can return the favor. By remaining a member of the group, you can help counsel others. You may even consider becoming a group leader. You can also help by making phone calls, sending out notices, and doing other routine chores. Most groups are run entirely by volunteers, so your help will be greatly appreciated. If you aren't a member of a group, you may want to start one. Scoliosis support groups offer a valuable community service.
>
> Another way to help others is through your doctor or hospital. Scoliosis specialists frequently ask teens who have worn braces or had surgery to talk

to others facing the experience. It doesn't take long—just a phone conversation or two—and you can really be a help. Sometimes all you have to do is listen.

Be an advocate. It is amazing how little is known about scoliosis. Research is needed to discover the cause (or, more likely, causes) of scoliosis, so that it can be treated more effectively. Also, we know scoliosis is genetic, but we don't know which genes are involved or what role they play.

The National Scoliosis Foundation and other scoliosis support groups help to raise money and consciousness for scoliosis research. If there are activities—such as races, bike-a-thons, or other events—in your community to raise money for scoliosis research, you can volunteer. If not, you may want to organize an event yourself. Local and national legislators need to be informed that this condition exists. Volunteers also work for more and better school screening programs, which promote early detection of scoliosis. At present, these programs are the best method of spotting scoliosis before complications have developed.

I started by saying this was a book about choices. These choices are yours and your family's to make. There's no right or wrong answer. Sometimes you may ask, "Why me?" That's okay, but only for a moment. With a positive attitude, and with a little help from your family, friends, and teachers, you'll come through with flying colors.

Glossary

A-P X rays X rays taken from front to back (anterior to posterior), with the patient standing and facing the X-ray machine. Lead shields are used to protect sensitive areas, such as breasts and reproductive organs, from radiation.

brace An external support of metal or plastic used to prevent scoliosis from progressing.

cervical vertebrae The seven vertebrae of the neck, which connect the thoracic (chest area) vertebrae with the skull.

Cobb angle Standard measure of scoliosis curves, named after the late Dr. John Cobb.

coccyx The four vertebrae at the bottom of the spine, which are fused together into a solid piece, also called the tailbone.

compensation The body's natural effort to keep the head centered over the pelvis and achieve balance throughout the length of the spine.

compensatory curve The body's effort to achieve compensation for a curve in one part of the spine by forming a smaller curve in the opposite direction in the other part. Sometimes called secondary curve.

CAT scan An abbreviation of computerized axial tomography, a form of X ray that produces cross-sectional images of internal structures, including the spine.

congenital Refers to any condition that is present at birth; not to be confused with *genetic.* Either heredity or trauma can produce a congenital abnormality.

decompensation A spinal imbalance in which the head is not centered over the pelvis.

disc A ring of cartilage with a soft, spongy core between two vertebrae in the spine.

distraction A method of correcting scoliosis by pulling the ends of the curve farther apart.

facet joints The joints that connect the vertebrae of the spine. They combine with discs to keep the spine strong and mobile.

fusion Joining individual vertebrae into a solid mass of bone by removing the material between them. The principal surgical technique used to correct scoliosis.

graft The process of transplanting tissue from one part of the body to another during surgery.

hardware Metal rods, screws, and wires used in scoliosis surgery to promote fusion and correct scoliosis during the healing process; can be removed if fusion is successful.

internal fixation A surgical technique that uses hardware to hold the spine straight after a fusion while the bone heals.

kyphosis The rounding of the upper part of the spine, when viewed from the side. Some degree of kyphosis is normal. Too much (humpback) is abnormal.

lordosis The front-to-back curve of the lowerpart of the spine, when viewed from the side. Too large a lordosis is called swayback. Lordosis, like kyphosis, can be flattened as a result of some treatments for scoliosis.

lumbar vertebrae The seven vertebrae of the lower back, between the thoracic spine and the sacrum.

MRI Magnetic resonance imaging, a diagnostic method that gives a three-dimensional view of internal structures, such as the spine, by use of a powerful magnetic field.

orthotist Someone who makes and fits orthopedic appliances, such as braces for scoliosis.

orthopedics The treatment of musculoskeletal disorders.

pedicles Oval indentations on the side of the vertebrae. When the pedicles move toward the midline, it is a sign that the vertebrae have rotated.

physiatrist A doctor who specializes in rehabilitation medicine.

pseudoarthrosis The failure of bone to fuse, sometimes occurring during surgery to correct scoliosis.

rib hump A protrusion of the ribs on one side of the back, caused by scoliosis and sometimes mistaken for abnormal kyphosis (humpback).

rotation A condition affecting the ribs, caused by the existence of a lateral curvature of the spine (scoliosis).

sacrum A piece of solid bone composed of five fused vertebrae between the coccyx (tailbone) and the lumbar or lower spine.

sagittal curve The natural curve of the spine when viewed from the side, resembling a gentle S shape. Too small a sagittal curve is called flatback.

scoliometer An instrument that when placed on the rib hump of a bending patient can measure degrees of rotation.

scoliosis A lateral (side-to-side) curvature of the spine.

spinal column The structure composed of vertebrae extending from the cranium (head) to the coccyx (tail) that encloses the spinal cord and forms the supporting axis of the body.

spinal cord The nerves encased within the spinal column. Part of the central nervous system.

thoracic vertebrae The twelve chest-area vertebrae that connect the lumbar spine to the neck or cervical spine and support the rib cage.

vertebrae Flexible pieces of bone that, connected by discs and facet joints, form the spinal column.

Where to Go for Help

Boston Brace, Inc.
20 Ledin Drive
Avon, MA 02322
tel: (800) 262-2235
fax: (800) 634-5048
e-mail: info@bostonbrace.com
Web site: http://www.bostonbrace.com
You can order specially made T-shirts designed to be worn under the Boston brace and other low-profile braces from this company.

The Feldenkrais Guild
524 Ellsworth Street SW
P. O. Box 489
Albany, OR 97321-0143
tel: (541) 926-0981
fax: (541) 926-0572
e-mail: feldngld@peak.org

Iyengar Yoga Institute
27 West 24th Street, Suite 800
New York, NY 10011
tel: (212) 691-9642; (800) 889-YOGA

National Scoliosis Foundation
5 Cabot Place

Stoughton, MA 02072
tel: (800) NSF-MYBACK [673-6922]
fax: (781) 341-8333
email: scoliosis@aol.com
The Foundation can provide you with useful information on all aspects of scoliosis diagnosis and treatment. It publishes a newsletter, *The Spinal Connection.*

The Pilates Studio®
2121Broadway, Suite 201
New York, NY 10023
tel: (212) 875-0189; (800) 474-5283
fax: (212) 769-2368
e-mail: MrPilates@aol.com
Web site: http://www.pilates-studio.com

The Scoliosis Association, Inc.
P. O. Box 811705
Boca Raton, FL 33481-1705
tel: (800) 800-0669

Scoliosis Research Society
6300 N. River Road
Suite 727
Rosemont, IL 60018-4226
tel: (847) 698-1627
fax: (847) 823-0536
Web site: http://www.srs.org

Shriners Hospitals for Crippled Children
Shriners Hospitals specialize in orthopedics for children. To locate the Shriners Hospital nearest you, call (800) 237-5055 in the United States or (800) 361-7256 in Canada.

For Further Reading

Barr, Linda. *Nothing Hurts but My Heart*. St. Petersburg, FL: Willowisp Press, 1995 (available from the National Scoliosis Foundation).

Blume, Judy. *Deenie*. New York: Bantam Doubleday Books for Young Readers, 1973.

Neuwirth, Michael, M.D., and Kevin Osborn. *The Scoliosis Handbook: A Consultation with a Specialist*. New York: Henry Holt and Co., 1996

Schommer, Nancy. *Stopping Scoliosis: The Complete Guide to Diagnosis and Treatment*. Garden City Park, NY: Avery Publishing Group, Inc., 1991 (available from the National Scoliosis Foundation).

Scoliosis Association, Inc. *Scoliosis*. Boca Raton, FL: Scoliosis Association, Inc., 1993.

Scoliosis Research Society. *Spinal Deformity: Scoliosis and Kyphosis—A Handbook for Patients*. Rosemont, IL: Scoliosis Research Society, 1995.

Shriners Hospital for Crippled Children, Chicago Unit. *Your Spinal Fusion Operation*. Chicago, IL: Shriners Hospital for Crippled Children, December 1994.

Videos

Growing Straighter and Stronger: Prescreening Education for Scoliosis, Grades 5–7. Available from the National Scoliosis Foundation.

Index